How I Survived Bone Cancer

Against All Odds

BARBARA J. MOCKFORD

How I Survived Bone Cancer
Copyright © 2012 by Barbara Mockford
www.facebook.com/The-Tri-Survivor
www.trisurvivor.nz
ISBN- 10: 1544262515
ISBN-13: 978-1544262512

This book is replicated from the original book called An Unshakeable Belief. I have just given this book a new book cover, title and subtitle

For Mum & Dad

Acknowledgements

I would like to acknowledge Automation Process & Control Group, Fonterra for their unwavering support; Paul Brown, Steve Hayward, and Ben Loveday for their strength to lean on during the hard times; Barbara and David Lee for their steadfast and resolute belief that I would prevail; Dr Gary French, my Doctor and friend, for saving my arm and keeping me sane; Dr Tom Palfi for keeping me fit, focused, and uncompromising; Dr Stewart Hardy for his honesty; Ward 25 and Ward 6 nurses at Waikato Hospital and the nurses at Manakau Super Clinic for helping me through the rough times; Lynne and Alan Taylor for bringing God into my Life; Wendy Chrisp for being my Ironman coach; Brad and Tracey Collins and Alma Tocker for being the kindest neighbours in a crisis; and Melissa Dobbs for being the best flatmate; Sam Caldwell for his assistance.

A special thanks to my friends for just being there for me: Kerry Suter and Gareth Drake, Anna Jones, Sarah Jenkins, Ruku I'Anson, Grant Budd, Wayne Reardon, Mike Reilly, Mike and Jane Gascoigne, Ian (Nobby) and Desiree McDonald, Kitzo, Mandy Moon, Grant Watters, Graeme Meyer, Steve MacIntyre, John Stanley, Philip and Marguerette Haycock, John Clark, Carl Gough, Paul Martin, James Lobb, Mike Fooy, Sherry Ludlam, Shane Wilkinson, Todd Preston, and Mary Gill; Danielle Nicholson for editing the first draft and her encouragement to finish this book.

A special thanks to Jay & Brooke Baker helping me Self Publish, it would not be possible without them.

My profound gratitude to my talented friend, Lauren Kim Roche, for her help and patience, which made this book possible. You encouraged me to never give up. See Lauren's book Bent Not Broken at BentNotBrokenBook.com

Lastly and foremost, thanks to Gael my beautiful Sister helping me through just everything and my loving family, I would not have gotten through this without you.

Table of Contents

Taupo Half Ironman

Dawn is just breaking and the mist is slowly lifting off the lake. The stars are fading into the light of day as I wheel my bike and gear into the transition area for today's triathlon. This is where we will change from wetsuits into bike clothes, then bike clothes into running gear. Quick transitions are important, as is discreetly discarding gear without flashing the other athletes and their families.

It is 5:30 a.m. I am the first competitor to arrive and I am a bundle of nerves. It is freezing cold and I am chilled to the bone. I stand my bike in the rack, then walk down to the edge of the lake. Silence and tranquillity surrounds me; the only noise is the ripple of wavelets finishing their journey as they ruffle the lake edge and sift watery fingers through hundreds of tiny, smooth pebbles. The scent of the gum trees around the car park is calming, reminding me of my childhood home and happy times. I remember making a hut in the gums with my kid brother on the farm. Finding a rock to sit on, I look across the distance where the sunrise has painted Mt. Ruapehu's snow-capped peak in shades of pink fading to an icy white blue. The magic of Lake Taupo is palpable.

In my mind, I hear the pre-race sounds of previous Ironman triathlons—the haka challenge—chanting Tuwharetoa Maori paddling their waka along the lakefront, the 1000-odd wetsuited competitors slowly entering the water. Competitors come from New Zealand, the Americas, Australia, Japan and up to thirty other countries. The music pumps over the P.A. system. Supporters line the edge of the lake cheering and clapping. The countdown begins, "Ten, nine, eight, seven," and Mike Reilly's voice booms out across the lake, giving encouragement and retelling the story of the Ironman.

"It all began in 1978 when 15 Marines argued over who was the strongest and fittest: swimmers, runners or cyclists. Over some drinks, they came up with the idea to put them all together in one stupendous race. On a beach in Hawaii, the marines combined several races already in existence and decided on a 3.8 km swim, a 180 km bike ride and a 42 km run. Each year, the challenge was taken up again and became known as the 'Ironman.'"

Every year, Mike's words roar out from his megaphone letting the athletes know how wonderful they are, telling them, "The days and months of training through wind, rain, sun and snow have been worth all the pain to be here on the start line. By the end of the day you will be AN IRONMAN!"

I am standing in the place where these words were spoken, these dreams begun. On the first Saturday of every March, Ironman New Zealand starts right here. The wind sighs in the pines. The crunch of tires on gravel reminds me others are arriving. Race time is an hour away.

This time yesterday morning I was still in bed, in my three-bedroom brick home in the city of Hamilton. My house has a lovely, large lounge with huge windows that catch the morning and afternoon sun. I often stand at the opening of the large French doors, look out at my neighbours and subdue winter's chill with the comforting heat from my fireplace. Hamilton is in the middle of the North Island of New Zealand, approximately 120 kilometres south of Auckland. I drove here in my Mazda MX5, adorned with my bike securely mounted on the tow bar. I have come to believe my MX5 is unique to NZ. I have logged many miles driving to events over the past several months and have never spotted another similarly accessorized Mazda.

It is now 5:45 Saturday morning and I am about to attempt my first Half Ironman. In eleven weeks, I will line up here with over a thousand others to tackle Ironman New Zealand. I will be an Iron virgin—tackling the full course for the first time. I have severe rheumatoid arthritis. My joints are painful and deformed, affecting all three disciplines of the triathlon. My audacity astounds my coaches, my family and me.

As I look along the lakefront, a bitter wind curls around me sending shivers down my back. Pulling my coat closer, I think it is going to be an icy cold swim. I smell a hint of rain in the air. Leaning down into the water and checking its temperature with my fingers reinforces my belief it's going to be a crazy day. What the hell am I thinking—swimming two kilometres at 6:30 a.m. in the freezing snowmelt that dribbles down from the mountains far on the other side of the lake? The wetsuit will help a bit, but it is still going to be the coldest swim of my life.

I look south of the start line, past the Taupo yacht club. Lights sparkle through the trees lining the lakefront road, a diamond necklace made from the homes and hotels that curl around the lake, reflecting and twinkling in the water. Later, along the same road, there will be people scattered around, watching the swim as well as the final run home. The footpath will be littered with posters of support from families patiently waiting to cheer their loved ones to the finish.

This Half Ironman follows the course of the full Ironman event in March, but is only half the distances: a 2 km swim, 90 km cycle and 21 km run. Walking back from the edge of the lake to transition, I double-check the gear I have set out for the bike and run, making sure I have all I could possibly need, placed in its correct order. Setting up transition is a ritual, offered to the gods of triathlon: the gods of lake and road, of no flat-tires, of a steady tail wind, any gods able to get the tired athlete home.

Slowly, one by one, competitors are arriving, loading their bikes on the racks at transition, checking all their gear and pulling on their wetsuits. As I look around at everyone, I see supremely fit looking people, relaxed and chatting to each other, catching up since they met at their last event. They look so relaxed, as if it was just another day at the office, unlike me attempting my first Half Ironman. What in the hell was I thinking? I kept reminding myself that triathletes like a person having a go. It does not matter what place you finish at or how good or bad you are. It is the mere fact of giving it a go; no one is a loser in a triathlon.

Indeed, it is a very democratic sport, where world champions routinely line up with novices. Just up from the lake edge, where we will get out of the water from the 2 km swim, there is a tent with two huge industrial gas heaters to warm us up after the swim and coax our frozen muscles into readiness for ninety kilometres of cycling. The water is so cold that wetsuits are compulsory. Any athlete not out of the water in seventy minutes will not be allowed to finish the race. The risk of hypothermia is real, an added incentive to swim hard.

"Ten minutes everyone. You should have your wetsuit on. Time to think about getting in the lake to warm up." The announcement by Wayne Reardon, one of the Race Directors, rattled over the public address system. "Warm up in this melted ice?" I thought to myself. "Yeah right…" Even the obligatory nervous pee in the wetsuit won't feel warm for long today.

Back at the edge of the lake, my friend Grant helps pull my wetsuit sleeve up my arms. I just don't have the strength; my arthritis is particularly bad at the moment, especially in my left forearm. Finally, he gets my wetsuit zipped up, making sure my pull cord is placed correctly with the Velcro tab at the back of the neck. If it's not right, it will chafe and hurt. I repeat the favour for him. Damn my left wrist is sore…

Grant is one of the most supportive and influential people I know. He got me into this sport. He is a very outgoing guy and not shy to say what he thinks about my training, whether it is funny, stupid, or critical. He has competed in Ironman several times and always has an opinion on my training or nutrition or rest schedule. We sometimes argue, but his intention is always encouraging and supportive. He makes time to answer my questions, however basic, and gives me loads of advice.

I am glad he is doing this triathlon with me. Grant is someone I can chat with at the start line, someone who will say something funny to make me laugh and take away the nerves as we shiver out into the cold water to await the start gun.

Grant took me to watch the 2005 Ironman event in Taupo. It was the most inspirational and overwhelming event I had ever witnessed, especially the final hour. The experience of being there, witnessing the pain and agony, the tears and the joy, the excitement and the overwhelming sense of achievement, was so intense it warmed me like flames dancing in a fire.

The event had a profound effect on me and continues to inspire me. I cannot imagine anyone not being moved when watching the athletes running, walking, wobbling or crawling the last two hundred meters down the finishing chute under the glow from the overhead lights—the music pumping, the crowd singing, cheering, clapping, and then, hearing the ritual words of Mike Reilly roaring, "You are an IRONMAN!"

As we wait for the next competitor to arrive at the finish line, Mike encourages the crowd to keep singing with the music, creating an epic competitive atmosphere that only he could. Amongst all the jubilation, a competitor comes running, crawling, limping down the finishing chute and the crowd just goes crazy! Mike deafens the crowd with "You Are an IRONMAN!" as they cross the finish line. In recognition of the effort this race demands, the finishing tape is placed up anew for every competitor. The Ironman finish is something I will always remember. That night, I decided that someday I wanted to hear that magical mantra for myself. Training through rain and sleet, as my arthritis burned and my lungs ached, I imagined Mike saying to me, "Barbara Mockford—you are an Ironman!" My eyes filled with tears whenever I imagined those words. Without fanfare, my life course had changed. I too would be an Ironman!

"Nine minutes everyone. You should have done your stretching by now. Slowly make your way down to the water. 13 Celsius isn't that cold, you know," announced Wayne with a wry smile in his voice.

Everywhere around me, there is nervous excitement. Spectators are hugging and wishing good luck to friends and family members bracing to enter the freezing water. There was no one to cheer for me—no family or partner. I was taking on this race alone apart from my friend Grant, but this race was not about a partner or friend cheering me on, it was a personal goal to achieve, a step to tick off on the way to the main event next year. I would ask my family to watch me achieve the impossible: to witness me walk or wobble over the finish line at Ironman New Zealand in March 2007, to share my triumph and joy.

It is only minutes before the start now. My wrist has swollen over three centimetres in circumference and throbs with every heartbeat. I take an extra couple of painkillers. Grant and I begin walking to the lake edge. I flinch as I walk over the cold stony beach and the odd sharp pebble stabs my feet. My stomach is doing nervous somersaults. Grant's wife gives him a hug for good luck and wishes me all the best. In the back of my mind I go over the past eleven months—training through rain, wind and sun, the events I had completed—hoping all my preparation would get me to the finish line today.

This is my big day, a test to see if I can achieve my goal of completing the Ironman in eleven weeks. As I ease into the water, it bites into every nerve ending in my body. The water is so cold that I find it difficult to breathe easily. Around me, people are gasping with the chill and I hear the odd screech as someone hits the icy water.

I look at these fit athletes, placing goggles over their eyes, showing no signs of anxiety, only excitement and determination. If only I had an ounce of their confidence! The mere thought of swimming in this freezing water is just mad! No matter how fast I tread water, my thin wetsuit gives very little insulation and I am cold to the core. Everyone around me is chatting about other triathlons, relating funny stories and other experiences that help take their minds, and mine, off of the enormity of the event. I do not have any stories to tell yet, but at the next triathlon, I too will have a story to share with someone just as nervous as I am to help take their fears away.

I was first diagnosed with rheumatoid arthritis in 1997. I was 32 at the time and engaged to be married. My fiancé was not supportive, and I was questioning our engagement while working long hours and not getting a lot of rest. On the bus to work one morning, I noticed a red patch on the side of two knuckles on my right hand. I could not recall banging or scraping my fingers, and put them out of my mind. When they looked worse and felt achy the next day, I made an appointment to see my family doctor. I knew about arthritis. My mother suffered from it, but I never imagined that I might have it. The doctor took blood tests, but the results did not confirm arthritis. We assumed I had knocked the fingers, and that the pain would go away. A couple of months later, my shoulder felt like glass shavings were rolling around it each time I moved and I was breaking into a sweat from just putting my suit on for work each morning.

I could hardly walk in my high heels. My ankles and hips were painful, and I tried to keep the pain at bay by taking high doses of Voltaren. I agreed to another blood test. This test was positive—the diagnosis of rheumatoid arthritis was official.

My life at the time was full of stress. I had two jobs, was going to the gym daily, not eating well, and had no support from my fiancé with household chores. I think these stresses all combined to overload my body, fast-tracking the onset of my arthritis. My diagnosis failed to spark needed physical and emotional support from my fiancé. Life for him carried on as usual. I still had to clean the house and cook. A year later, I broke our engagement and left him. My arthritis continued to bring pain, but my personal life improved immensely.

Wayne's voice cuts through my reverie, "Five minutes everyone! You should be warmed up now. Start thinking about where you want to be on the start line, making sure you're in the right place. If this is your first big event or you are nervous swimming with others, sit at the back and let the others go ahead. Swim smart, pace yourself. Have a good day out there everyone! You have worked hard to be here today so enjoy the moment!"

He has to be kidding! How can anyone be enjoying this bloody cold water? All I can feel is pain! I put my face in the water and feel the beginnings of hyperventilation caused by the cold. I will have to concentrate on slow, deep breaths. I wonder if an ice cream headache will take my mind off my arthritic left wrist.

"Thirty seconds to go everyone! Have a great day! Be proud of getting to the start line and good luck!"

The only good thing about this water being so cold is that it numbs my wrist, which is now hideously swollen. Last night, I visited the hospital in Taupo to request a cortisone injection to settle the pain in my wrist. Because it was a small local hospital with minimal staffing, they declined. I hoped the combination of the painkillers I took at 4:30 this morning and the freezing water would give me some relief. I cannot believe that today of all days, my arthritis decides to have its own little party! Ignoring pain is normal for me, but today it is extra bothersome. I just have to try to ignore my wrist, which is now twice its normal size.

"Enjoy the race everyone! We will see you at the finish line!"

Bang!

Suddenly, I find myself among a flurry of seemingly disconnected arms and legs. The odd unintended kick in the face and choking mouthful of water remind me to stay focused. I decide to let everyone go on ahead and enjoy the moment. Setting a steady, slow pace, I ignore the irritation I begin to feel in my left arm. I just keep the right arm following the left arm round and round, concentrating on moving forward. I look up after five hundred meters, and notice that almost everyone is already going around the first buoy. They have gone nine hundred meters to my five hundred. It is a relief and wonderful feeling of achievement to reach the first buoy. After a short pause to congratulate myself, I realize I now

need to swim seventy meters across the lake to the second buoy before turning back towards the yacht club. Seventy meters, only three lengths of the training pool in my neighbourhood. I stop for a moment to catch my breath and get some respite from the freezing, crystal-clear lake water. I have never known my arthritis to hurt so much. Perhaps the adrenaline of the event is amplifying the pain.

I put my face back in the water and struggle to slow my breathing.

"Oh shit, I will never make it!"

Stay focused. "It's only arthritis, there are other folks going through worse pain in the world."

I finally reach the last buoy to head back to the finish when I realize someone is yelling at me.

"Hey, this way. Hey over there, this way. Hey you—this way!"

I stop swimming to look up. A race marshal on a surfboard is yelling at me and trying to get my attention. I am swimming in the wrong direction toward Mt. Ruapehu! If he had not yelled at me, I might be still swimming stroke by painful stroke toward the mountains. Swimming in the right direction during the last leg, I felt a searing, burning sensation in my left arm. I decide to try to swim with one arm, which is clearly unsuccessful. Even though the pain seems unbearable, I resign myself to using both arms while getting to the finish line. I kept saying to myself, "It's just arthritis. Get over it." I think I can manage this pain on the bike and the run. I just have

to make it to the shore.

Only a few months ago, I was on a beautiful island in Fiji swimming in 25° (77°F) water in a pool, with my sister Gael lounging poolside saying, "You look like a drowning turtle." How different it is now in the 13° (55°F) water of Lake Taupo. I must really look like a drowning turtle with only one arm engaging properly. Two hundred meters from the finish line, two race marshals are paddling along each side of me to guide me home. They are a bit close for my liking, so I temporarily stop swimming and tread water.

"Don't get too close to me please," I plead. I appreciate their attentiveness in guiding me to the finish line. It is wonderful, but I am so fearful that with my arms flailing around in this haphazard way I will hit their paddles. Still treading water, I said with a weak smile to the race marshals in the kayak and on the surfboard, "I'm worried I will hit my arm on your paddle. Could you paddle a bit further out from me? I've got bad arthritis and my arm is killing me."

"Yeah, sure, no problem. You have not got far to go now, just stop when you want to stop. We can help you onto the back of the kayak and get you into a warm tent to thaw out when you are back on shore." His demeanour was reassuring but I could hear concern in his voice.

"Thank you both, but I would like to finish this swim. I have to be able to say I at least finished the swim."

The race marshal on the surfboard said, "Hey don't worry about us. Take your time. We will be right beside you if you change your mind." Time was ticking by and the colder I got, the more I realized my day of racing was about to end.

I finally got out of the water second to last, being helped out by those fantastic men. I felt like a walking block of ice. They directed me into the first aid tent where two glorious gas heaters were running like jet engines blasting the cold out of me. The attendants carefully stripped my wetsuit off and wrapped me up in blankets. Sitting next to me was another competitor shivering and drinking hot chocolate. The smell of chocolate and the thought of drinking something so smooth, warm and comforting was divine. Next thing I knew I had one in my cold blue hands. The chocolate tasted great, but defeat left a bad taste on my lips.

"God I feel sick and my arm hurts like hell. It must be five centimetres bigger in circumference now." A medic in the tent was watching over the cold competitors.

"Have you taken any medication?"

"Yeah, all of my arthritis medication at 4:30, three Salazo-pyrin and two Paradex, then another couple of Paradex at 6:15."

"You have probably taken too much medication, which is making you feel nauseated."

"Mmm, it is the maximum amount prescribed for me, but you may be right. My arm is burning like hell!"

"See how you feel after you finish your hot chocolate and you are a bit warmer."

I look around outside the tent at all the spectators and can see my coach Wendy Chrisp among them, which is reassuring. Wendy walks up to the tent.

"Hey Barbs, how are you doing?"

"I feel terrible Wendy, my arm hurts like hell! I feel sick and there is no way I can carry on with the bike and run. It's gutting after all our hard work."

"Come back to my place and have a hot shower and change and we will chat about where we go from here, okay?"

Wendy stayed with me in the tent until I was feeling warm, less sick, and able to drive back to her house to refresh myself. The rest of the day was a write-off. Firstly, I was frozen. Secondly, my arm was agonizing. And thirdly, I was terribly nauseated. The race medic was probably right. I had taken too many painkillers—so I ended up sitting on the main street cheering for the other athletes while munching on McDonald's and hoping the food would settle my stomach.

The odds of a spot prize in this race are good as there are only about 150 competitors. I mentioned to my coach that at least I completed the swim and would not feel too guilty if I won a spot prize. It was frustrating seeing everybody finish, smiles of jubilation on their tired faces, the finishers' medal hung around their necks, their friends and family running up to congratulate them. I was happy for the finishers, but heartbroken I did not have the same experience and result.

For the past eleven months, I had trained like a robot: completing each week's training with a report for my coach, completing the 100 km cycle race from Rotorua to Taupo, the half-marathon in Taupo, an 80 km leg of the 160 km cycle race around Lake Taupo, and the Tinman triathlon at Mt. Maunganui.

Today, I was putting all my training together to test my ability to attempt the full Ironman. On a positive note, in a couple of weeks I would be back in training, assuming my arthritis settles down. I could get a cortisone injection in the painful area in my arm and test myself at the Rotorua Half Ironman next Saturday with my friend, Lauren.

Lauren Roche is a doctor, author and friend I made at one of the training camps our coach, Wendy, organized in the middle of the year in Taupo. On one of the rest days, Lauren and I went to a cafe for lunch to swap notes, grouch about training and commiserate on all the things we miss out on during the weekends while we are out on the road cycling or training in the other two disciplines.

Lauren lives in Napier and was attempting her first Ironman in 2007. She has so much spunk; short, short blond hair; pink-rimmed glasses; and a gorgeous sports car. Hearing her story of riding her stationary cycle a hundred meters down her hillside garden while training inspired me even more to pursue my crazy idea to do an Ironman. Lauren loves everything pink. I could not stop smiling after she told me she was going to wear pink shoes, pink skirt, pink top, pink cap, pink everything at next week's Half Ironman in Rotorua.

Despite only completing the swim leg, I won a triathlon wetsuit from one of the event sponsors, Xterra! The wetsuit was beautiful, smooth and soft like a second skin. I was so excited about winning that I left my $300 sunglasses on a table at the prize giving. Realizing my loss several minutes later, I raced back to thankfully find them still there! What a relief that was.

Driving back home to Hamilton, my pain was horrific. Anyone following me would probably have thought I was drunk! I drove with one arm and found fifth gear very difficult to manage. Grant and his wife followed me. A quick stop for a coffee in a small town on the way home gave me five minutes to relax. I looked at Grant through my car window and said, "God my arm is still bloody sore! I can hardly drive!"

"Toughen up B, it's only an arm."

"Yeah right. You drive with a sore arm and nausea. If it was you, a bloke, you would act as though the world was coming to an end."

"Pain is your friend B." Grant had two mantras while road cycling, "pain is your friend" and "hills are your friend." I didn't believe either of those monstrous lies.

"Yeah, yeah, bleat, bleat, bleat."

Grant smiled at my remark and closed his car door.

That night I was still feeling ill and at one point raced to the bathroom, only to dry retch. I had a pitiful night's sleep. I woke up feeling nauseated and rushed to the bathroom again to dry retch. I knew this was not a normal arthritis symptom.

I walked into my flatmates' room, showing them my swollen wrist. (I lived with a cardiac nurse, Mel, and her friend, also a nurse.) They felt I needed urgent medical assessment. I rang Mum and told her. She agreed that I should go to the hospital, so I did.

The usual wait in the Emergency Department was terrible. It was just after nine on a Sunday morning; I wanted to get out of this place, full of crying babies and the groans of the sick and injured. Finally, a nurse called my name and walked me through to the Emergency section of the clinic for an X-ray.

Back in my cubicle, the attending doctor put the X-ray up on the light box. I knew a little about X-rays from the many I had taken for arthritis checks on my joints. He stood back to examine it. I do not need the doctor to tell me that my wrist is broken. The bones do not line up properly, and, more worrisome, there is a large black spot where crisp white bone should be. I know straight away that my bone is not normal.

A frown appeared on the doctor's face. He had taken my medical history earlier and knew that I was quite fit. He looked worried and puzzled. He went away with my X-ray to consult with his colleagues. In the meantime, I rang Mum and gave her an update.

I fractured the radius in my left forearm while I was doing the Half Ironman swim, explaining that hot, burning sensation and subsequent increase in pain. The black patch on my radius freaked me out the most. I did not want to think too hard about what it might mean.

While waiting for Mum, Gael and the doctor, I rang my brother Allan to wish him a happy birthday. I told him that I was in the hospital with a broken arm and a black spot on one of the bones. Allan is not someone who chats for long on the phone, only necessary information

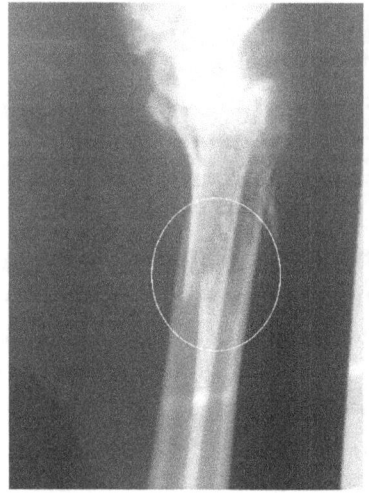 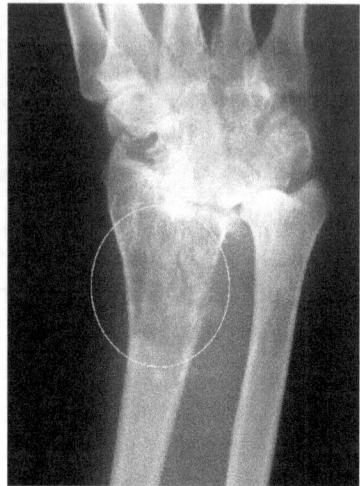

Fractured Left Radial　　　*Tumour on Radial (dark spot)*

is shared before he ends the call. I said goodbye and assured him I would call him the next day.

Gael and Mum arrived. The doctor put the X-rays back on the display wall and pointed to the black patch on my left radius. He felt it was probably infected. The radius looked like a tree with a rotten branch. Osteomyelitis, an infection in the bone, was the probable diagnosis. Such an infection would cause a weak spot that appeared black on an X-ray.

The doctor suggested the mechanical stresses of a long swim could easily make the weakened bone splinter.

To confirm his diagnosis, the doctor took a bone biopsy. He covered my skin with topical anaesthetic for 45 minutes, and then injected a local anaesthetic in the same place. When he brought out another syringe, my jaw dropped—the needle was so long! The doctor told me he had to push this long needle through my bone and suck out bone marrow to do cultures to determine what bug I had.

Looking at the long needle going into my wrist made me feel sick. I absolutely hate needles! I could feel the pressure of the needle on my bone. The resistance offered by the bone forced the doctor to gradually guide the needle through my swollen wrist and made the procedure seem excruciatingly slow. It was a heavy, dull feeling rather than pain. I wanted it all to be finished quickly but it was like watching a horror film in slow motion. It took an absolute eternity for the syringe to fill with marrow. All the way through the procedure, my doctor said supportive words and commented on how brave I was. I was all alone apart from the doctor. Gael and Mum had driven home to Te Awamutu, a 40 minute drive away. Mum was worn out, as she also suffers severe arthritis and tires easily. I was glad they did not witness this awful procedure; it would have been horrible for them both.

The doctor admitted me to the hospital overnight, waiting for the culture results. Lying in my bed, I realized there was no chance I would be able to do the Rotorua Half Ironman the following Saturday with Lauren. That sucked. Not to be disappointed, I decided the next best thing would be to become her support crew and cheer her home during the long swim, cycle race and run around Blue Lake. I planned my escape from the hospital on Friday. I would buy pink pom-poms and anything else pink that I could find to wave and cheer for my Iron buddy. Feeling a lot happier with a plan and loads of fun to look forward to, I was able to drift off to sleep, confident that when I awoke the doctors would surely tell me I could leave after a couple of days of antibiotics to cure the infection in my arm.

My reality was different. The next morning during ward rounds, the doctors said I needed to have more tests run over the next three days. I thought it was strange to be having a chest X-ray and a CT scan of my abdomen, followed by MRI scans, as well as a full body bone scan. It seemed like overkill for a bug in my arm.

Thursday morning the doctors came round for their usual discussions about my arm. When they had finished, I told them I needed to discharge myself the next day to drive down to Rotorua to be support crew for Lauren's Half Ironman. They agreed this was okay after they put my arm in a plaster cast—luckily, the plaster room had fluorescent pink. . It looked so happy! Lauren would be most impressed.

The doctors agreed I could have a weekend pass on the proviso that I checked back into the hospital on Monday morning.

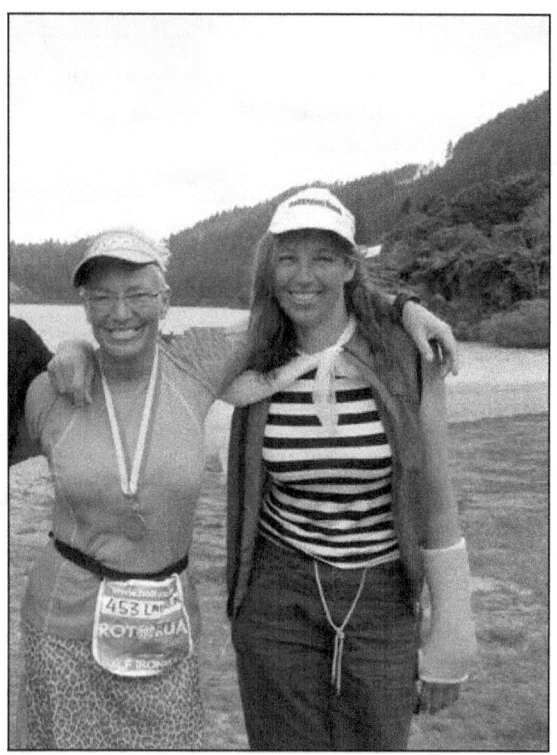

Lauren Roche and I (with my Pink Cast)

Tea And A Chaplin

Lauren did really well! She had a panic attack in the swim, walked for the steepest uphill parts of the bike race and finished near the back of the field, but managed to smile all the way. I cheered her on waving pink pom-poms! It was loads of fun supporting her and the other competitors. With great reluctance, I checked back in to Waikato Hospital on the 18th of December for another biopsy of the black spot on my radius.

Two days later during the morning doctors' rounds, I questioned them about the second biopsy, asking what they found wrong with the bone. The doctors said they did not take out any bone but some flesh of some description, which I thought very strange. The doctors' visits were so fast that I could never remember all the questions I had in my mind while they were furiously discussing me with each other. After they left, I rang Mum. Unable to answer all of her questions, I realized I had no idea what was going on, so I asked a nurse to have one of the doctors come back and explain the biopsy in more detail. I needed to find out what was actually biopsied and why. My mum needed answers and so did I.

I waited for the doctor in the TV lounge. I was dressed in a t-shirt and jeans—I hated staying in the hospital nightshirts. I wasn't sick and I didn't want to be turned into a patient. I was Barb, and until recently, I had been training to be an Ironman. How could I be sick?

Ten minutes later, the young doctor arrived.

"What tissue did you cut out of my arm?" I asked. There was a long silence. He looked at his shoes, then out the window before looking at me in a very empathetic way, which made my stomach drop.

"A small piece of a tumour."

"A what? I thought it was infected bone you were checking." I hoped I had heard wrong. Nurses were going up and down the ward. The TV was manic with a morning show. All of this noise slowly faded into the background after I heard the word "tumour."

"No. We found a lump on top of the bone, the size of an old 20c piece," he said. As he glanced down at his shoes, I thought how young, caring and uncomfortably out of his depth he seemed.

"When will I know what kind?" I asked quite remotely.

"The results will be back on the 28th of December." He inspected his shoes again, "Would you like me to get the chaplain for you?"

"No thanks." Why would I want a chaplain who was a stranger and did not know me at all? If the chaplain looked like Pierce Brosnan that would be ok but it still would not change what I had just heard. We talk about my bone, about results—and then jump straight to the chaplain! The doctors must be really worried. I was learning that hospitals have two answers for distress—a nice cup of tea, or the chaplain.

The young doctor left with a sad look on his face. I was all alone. I felt an awful sinking feeling in the bottom of my gut.

I cannot believe this is happening to me! I forced back the lump in my throat, followed by a heavy swallow. Fear was slowly clouding my mind as I considered the word "tumour." Nothing about that word was positive. Nothing about my thoughts was comforting or good. I tried to shut those thoughts away and slowly let what the doctor told me trickle through my mind. I needed to contact Mum and Dad.

Mum answered the phone. In a semi-cheerful tone I said, "Hello, Mommy," in the posh English way I learned when I stayed with friends in England. Their daughter always said "Mommy" in such a groovy way that from time to time I say it like her for a giggle. I needed a giggle, but wasn't sure I would ever have a genuine one again.

"Hi. What did the doctor say?"

"He said I had a tumour," I say in a very strong "I am okay" voice.

"Oh shit."

"It's okay, Mum, they don't know what sort and hey, it's probably benign." My voice managed to sound upbeat and cheerful.

"Okay then. You ring me anytime you feel the need to talk."

Staying strong and with a smile in my voice for Mum I said, "Yip, okay."

I really felt bad about calling Mum. I did not want to burden her with this news as she has her own health issues and Grandma was not well. My health was the last thing I wanted Mum to worry about, but she would be more upset if I did not tell her.

On the brink of tears, I sent a text with my awful news to Kerry, my mate and work colleague, and almost started crying. I did not get an immediate reply, but I knew he would contact me soon. I thought, "Now I am not going to cry—tears never solve, fix or change anything."

I was struggling to keep myself from weeping. I forced the muscles of my eyelids to quickly close and open a couple of times, hoping this would stop any further tears. I felt my eyes welling up. They were red and stinging. My traitorous wrist ached and burned too.

I thought of Mum and Dad, and wondered what Dad would be saying right now. I could hear him, "Crying isn't going to help or make any difference to the situation." He was right. I told myself to suck it up while my eyes were burning in pain, begging to cry, but I just held it in.

My dad has made me very independent. I was taught to rely only on myself when the going gets tough. Dad spoke words of sense and logic when I went through rough times, either at school when I was young or through challenging times as an adult. I did not know any different growing up. He has made me strong and self-reliant, qualities I have called on again and again in my Ironman training and would need in spades in my new battle for my health.

I thought, "God, this sucks, this is not fair!" A tear tracked down my face and I mentally told myself off. I looked out the hospital window over Hamilton, thinking of all the people out there working—people on holiday, people worrying about day-to-day things, stressed at work, hating work, enjoying work, giving birth, laughing, training—wishing I were one of those people. I looked out the window from the hospital lounge at the city, all the office buildings, the yachts on the lake, the hills in the distance, the trees amongst the houses and the buildings surrounding the lake. My eyes wandered down the Waikato River and I thought how beautiful Hamilton is. The cars driving up the hill, where were they going? Why could I not be in one of those cars going somewhere, my mind on all of the things I would rather be thinking about, or doing, or worrying about, than what I am thinking now?

The nurses saw me looking upset and one asked, "Would you like to see a chaplain?"

"No thanks."

I was trying hard not to sound exasperated, knowing they were doing their best to make me feel better about things. "What can a chaplain do?" I wanted to shout at them. What I really wanted was a friend to be with me. However, they were all working and I did not want to bother them. I gave in and texted Kerry again.

The texts I received from Kerry cheered me up. I think I even rang him for a minute or so. I can't quite remember, as that whole hour is a blur. Questions were haphazardly going through my mind like a checklist. Was it this? Was it that? Was the tumour caused by hours and hours of training? Was my immune system deficient? It did not make sense. I desperately wanted a cause. I needed a reason. If something I had done had caused this, perhaps there was something I could do to fix it.

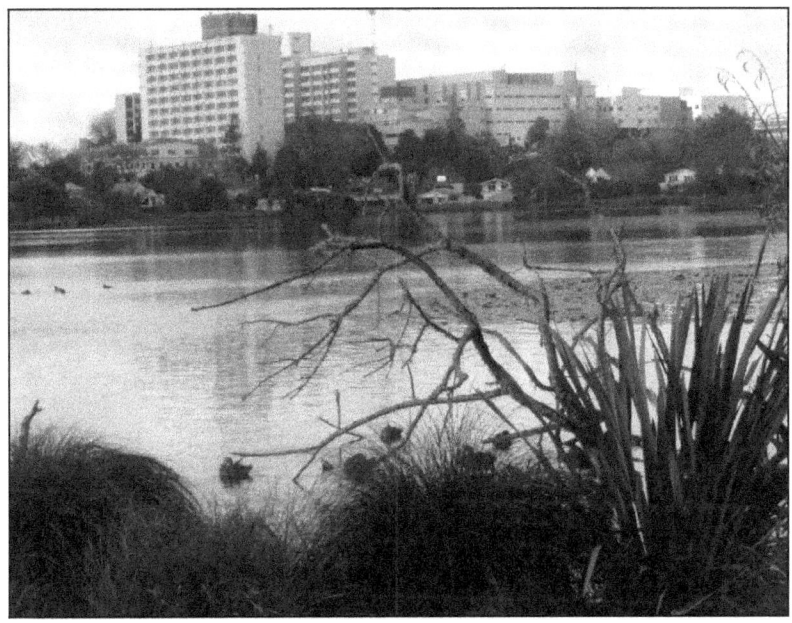

Waikato Hospital

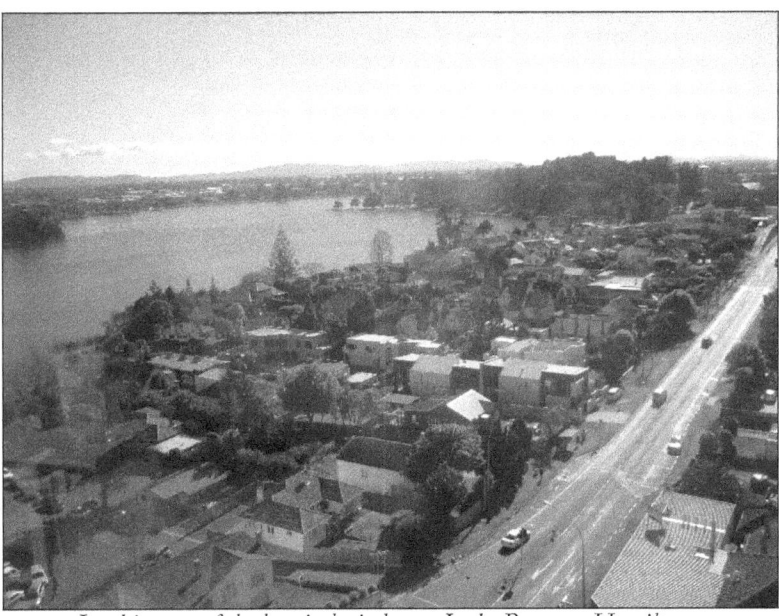

Looking out of the hospital window at Lake Rotoroa, Hamilton

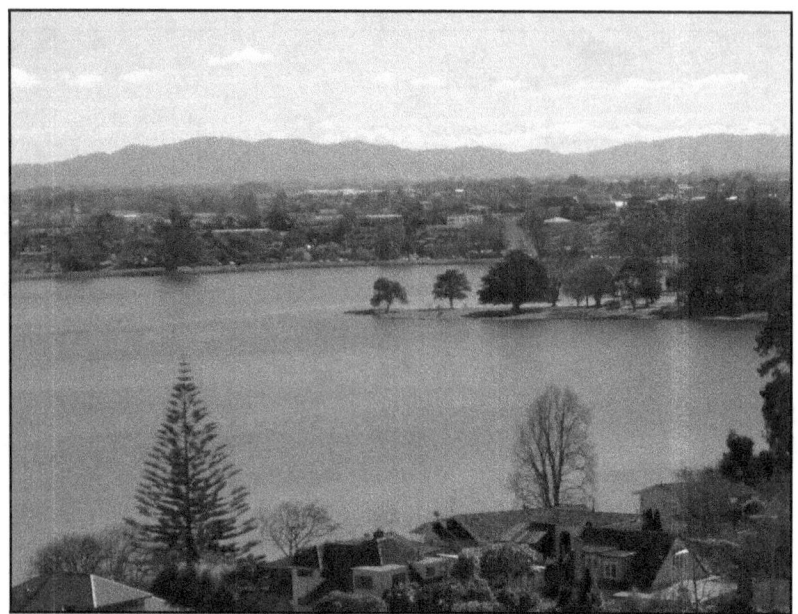

Looking out of the hospital window at Lake Rotoroa, Hamilton

What Had I Done

I thought back over the past eleven months, wondering if there was anything I had done wrong to get a tumour. Before I began the training required for Ironman, I consulted a nutritionist and made sure my diet was right. I went to a physiotherapist to check my core muscle strength. I hired a professional coach. I had blood tests. I went to my doctor making sure what I had planned was okay. My doctor friend, Tom, said this event was "doable." I was often told by friends that I was spending too much money on professionals, but I was determined to do everything right.

I ate like a rugby player. My plate was enormous every night. I had steak or meat of some kind, with huge amounts of mashed potatoes and vegetables. I invested in whey protein powder to facilitate the repair and growth of muscles. I rested when I needed to, knowing that recovery was one of the cornerstones of training. No matter how much I was eating and resting, though, I was always tired. I could never work that out. I remembered telling my coach, "I need two weeks to taper, to build up energy for the Half Ironman event."

When she agreed, it felt like a huge holiday.

Unfortunately, on race day, I still did not feel 100%. I blamed my arthritis.

What bothered me the most was that I would not be going over the 2007 Taupo Ironman finish line. I would not hear Mike Reilly say, "Barbara Mockford: You. Are. An. IRONMAN!"

I had worked so hard and focused on this big day for so long. Wiping another tear from my cheek, I focused on the positive side—at least I could go to Ironman as a volunteer. I could still be part of the event, learn what happens inside the large tent adjacent to the finish line and share the glory of watching my friends finish. This gave me something to look forward to and helped distract me from my heartbreak.

I also remembered I had a Half Ironman to do in January as part of a team. I was the swimmer, Shane Wilkinson was the cyclist and Sarah Jenkins was the runner. Oh my God.

"How am I going to swim with a cast on?" I asked myself and laughed.

Kerry came to mind straight away, as he is an excellent swimmer. I sent him a text to see if he was free on the 6th of January 2007 to do the swim section of the Half Ironman for me.

Kerry sent a text back and replied that he would be down on the South Island tramping. I decided I had to do it. It had cost me a lot to enter and I had a good incentive to do this event. The only possible section of this triathlon I could complete was the run. There was no way I could swim or cycle with my wrist in plaster. Excited by this decision, I sent off texts to Sarah and Shane asking if we could swap the team around. I asked Shane if he could do the swim and Sarah the cycling. I would do the run instead of Shane, but of course I would walk the half-marathon. They agreed with no reservations. That quickly got my mind to focus on my strategy to walk a half-marathon. It was only fifteen days until race day at Mt. Maunganui. I felt myself going forward, not letting the heart-breaking news of my possible cancer override my usual optimism.

I was discharged from the hospital, awaiting the results of the recent biopsy. This gave me time to get some walking training done before the Tauranga Half Ironman run leg.

I made a call to Steve, my manager at work, to let him know that I had a tumour on my left arm. My doctor advised me that I would be off work for two weeks. Being away from work this long did not feel right, nor did conveying the bad news to Steve. During my conversation with Steve, he asked me if I had read Lance Armstrong's book *It's Not About the Bike: My Journey Back to Life*.

I said, "No. What's it about?"

"Lance tells how he got through testicular cancer and went on to become such a great athlete. It's a brilliant read. Later on today I will buy it for you and bring it in when I see you tomorrow."

"Thanks! Bring in any work that I can do, too," I said with a smile.

"You just worry about getting well. Do not worry about work, it will still be here when you get back." I could feel Steve's sincere concern and kindness as he spoke. His simple offer to gift the book gave me a needed boost and helped me refocus on all that was good in my life.

I mentally reviewed the past twelve months again and tried to figure out if I had done anything stupid which could have caused the tumour. Thoughts of "if only I" or "what if I" kept eating away at me. What really puzzled me was I thought I would feel fit after training six months, even with arthritis. I was so irritated with not having any bounce in my step. I was always so exhausted and resigned myself to the fact that it was my arthritis. Arthritis, by its painful nature, drains your energy, even if you are not exercising. Being tired was just something I had become used to, even expected. I now realized that my tiredness might have been a bad sign I had innocently ignored.

Thinking back to the two kilometre swim last Saturday, the pain in my arm made sense.

At least there was no sign the tumour had spread beyond the bone. Cancer shifts from its original (primary) site to distant places in the body through the blood or lymphatic systems and the cells grow as secondary cancers or metastases. The good news was that my CT, body scans and other X-rays were clear. There were no metastases from the cancer seen in my abdomen, lymph nodes, lungs and vital organs. This was the only good news my doctors had to give me, and I clung to it.

On the 28th of December, Gael came with me to my appointment to meet my orthopaedic surgeon, Dr Hardy. We were to find out the results of my biopsy. I arrived early just as I had at the Half Ironman a few weeks ago in Taupo, except this time my sister was with me. Gael is a policewoman—clear-headed and strong in difficult situations.

Dr Hardy met us after his ward rounds.

After the introductions, his first comment was, "The hospital lab was unable to give a definitive result from your biopsy. We have sent some of your tissue to Auckland Hospital to get the diagnosis."

I sat there in a daze and let Gael ask all the questions. In her authoritative voice she asked, "Is the radius the primary site?"

"Yes, it is. Auckland Hospital should have the full results by the 15th of January."

"What does primary mean?" I asked, having never heard of this term before.

"It's the place where the cancer started," Gael said.

"Oh," I said, none the wiser, and decided to quiz Gael on the way home.

Gael is very good at asking all the right questions and giving all the right answers. She is able to listen to the medical mumbo jumbo, analyse what is pertinent, and fire back a difficult question when needed. Every sick person needs an advocate like her. I enjoyed listening to her debating issues with Dr Hardy, seeing the appreciation on his face, being able to discuss a difficult issue with someone who understood exactly what he was saying, and who did not get emotional or angry. Her focus made for a short and concise meeting.

There was no way I would remember the guts of this meeting with the doctor. I knew Gael would. On the way home, she translated the whole discussion in a way that I was able to understand. This did not make me feel any better, but at least I knew what my situation was medically. It's easier to fight an enemy when you have some understanding of it.

I was furious and frustrated. Of all the time to wait for results! Christmas and New Year's means the whole country almost stops. Nearly everybody goes to the beach. The most difficult part of this nightmare was not being in control and having to wait to have the tumour identified before it could be removed from my body to prevent it from growing further. The parasite was able to have its own Christmas holiday and continue its merry life for another three to four weeks, free to invade more of my bone and do other sinister things! The tumour had desires to fulfil, and I was its unwilling host till the holiday season was over.

I went back to work in between Christmas and New Year's Eve, which took my mind off things a bit. I was an administrator and typist for Fonterra, at the Te Rapa Dairy Factory. I updated and distributed Quality Manuals, retyped accrediting standards, relieved reception, and coordinated national and international travel for staff. When there were quiet patches, my imagination took over and I became morose, wondering if the tumour was growing and spreading. On occasion, I would just stare out the window for ages trying to escape reality. At times I would get up from my desk and walk down to visit my workmates in Systems.

The Systems department looked after all the automated computer systems in all the different Fonterra sites around New Zealand. I walked down the corridor to their office to see how their day was going and inject some lightness into mine. We would chat about the music they had playing, or the latest movie, or other topics of the moment. Sometimes, I would just walk to their office to sit and listen to all of their conversations to take my mind off things. It was always enjoyable there, with lots of hilarity and teasing. It was a great place to escape my morbid thoughts, and be amongst merriment.

January 2007 Tauranga

Sarah and I left Hamilton at five in the morning headed for the Port of Tauranga and the Half Ironman meet at Mt. Maunganui. Shane was already there having spent the New Year's holiday in Tauranga with his family. The triathlon started at seven, with Shane swimming against the tide during half of the race. The water was cold and he was glad to finish, running to meet Sarah in transition, so she could cycle ninety kilometres around the streets of Mt. Maunganui.

True to my commitment to Lauren, I was sporting a pink cast. I did not bother about a sling—it would only get in my way. While I was waiting for Sarah in transition, a race marshal came round and sprayed us all with a sponsor's sunblock. It was a boiling hot, sunny day, and the sunscreen lotion was a welcome relief. Sarah soon came into transition, glad to get off her bike, so I could start the half-marathon run.

Walking the run section had been the plan from day one for my triathlons, including the Ironman's 42 kilometre run. I could not believe how long the twenty-one kilometres was taking me and what made it worse was the blistering heat. The cut off time for the event was one in the afternoon. At one o'clock in the afternoon I don't think I was even a quarter of the way around the first 10.5 kilometre lap. This did not worry me. I was doing my own little race. Pacing myself, I was slowly working out how long it would take to complete a full marathon in future Ironman events. I was Tail End Charlie. A race marshal's vehicle drove in front of me at a snail's pace, with yellow flashing lights mounted on the roof warning traffic.

I felt like a hazard to oncoming traffic and found it slightly embarrassing. For a few moments I entertained the idea that I was a VIP with someone in front saying, "Make way please," creating space for me to walk through crowds of people. That thought did not last long. I was still racing and it was quite embarrassing, really. The whole event had finished three hours ago. I was still trying to get to the finish line, walking along the ocean front road, sweat dripping off of me, sporting a pink cast. At one house I past, there was a group of people on the balcony having a nice cold beer. One of the guys yelled out, "Would you like a beer?"

"Hell yes!"

"C'mon up and get one."

"Sure, when I've finished this race."

Stopping would have been in violation of racing rules punishable by instant disqualification. With a distant reward of a cold beer firmly planted in my mind, I walked on along the never-ending road, focused on the mountain in front of me. Just before I walked around the base of Mt. Maunganui, I had to pass all the shops and cafes. There were loads of people sitting at tables having cold drinks and food. At the time it seemed like cruel and unusual punishment hearing their laughter and enjoyment while I sweltered in the sun.

As I came round the mountain and walked down the hill back onto the road, the race marshal's vehicle (along with Shane and Sarah, my friends and fellow competitors, and Sherry and her husband) was waiting for me. Cheers and shouts of support motivated me to keep going. I was so inspired by their support. In the last hundred meters to the finish line their clapping inspired me to find the last remnants of energy that remained in my body, and I managed to run over the finish line. It was the least I could do, to show respect for my friends, as well as the event. What a surprise and encouragement is was to find that the organizers of the event had left the "finish" sign mounted on the frame over the finish line. The best surprise was that the director of the Port of Tauranga race was waiting for me. He said I deserved the finishers' medal that he put around my neck, for the sheer fact of not giving up. I could not believe this important man waited for me; it was so humbling.

On the 10th of January, I received a call from Dr Hardy asking me to pop in for another biopsy on the 16th of January. Waikato

Hospital was cranking back into life with staff back from their two week holiday. It had been a long, glorious summer and the place was gearing up for another demanding, hectic year. Dr Hardy told me that Auckland hospital required more of my tumour for further tests. This was not encouraging.

The operation was more painful than the biopsy in December. I decided to go for all the painkillers they offered: morphine was first, followed by tramadol. I found tramadol frightening and just plain horrible as it gave me side effects of nausea, dizziness and depersonalization. In the future, this painkiller is definitely on the "Do Not Use" list for me. Never again would I entertain the idea of tramadol no matter how much pain I was in.

The next morning during doctor's rounds, Dr Hardy told me told that I should get the results of this biopsy by the end of January. Just before he and his entourage of doctors and nurses left my room, he nonchalantly said, "Be prepared to lose your arm."

"Where, err where will it be cut off?"

"About here," he said pointing to just below my left shoulder.

At first, I thought he was joking, but the look of his face and the tone of his voice did not fit with a joke. I felt he knew more than he was letting on. The nurses quickly came back, aghast from the delivery of his announcement. I was totally devastated and shocked by his manner, and wanted to strangle him with said arm. I looked at the nurses and saw the empathy on their faces and quickly said, "No, no chaplain, please. I am going to get out of bed, walk down the hall, and make a strong, sweet coffee. Keep the chaplain in his church this time."

I sat in the most comfortable chair in the TV lounge looking out the picture window and sipping on almost toffee sweet coffee. I was thinking about how things just kept getting worse. I did a mental summation: almost getting hit with a paddle; swimming with a broken arm; a tumour, not the expected and more benign arthritic inflammation; being asked if I wanted a chaplain; and now, the possible amputation of my left arm!

I rang one of my friends who had a great sense of humour. He told me all the positive things there were about having one arm, which made me laugh. Gloves would be cheaper, my nail polish bottles would last twice as long, no one would expect me to type quickly… It snapped me out of my doom and gloom mood and forced me to look forward. Soon I would have a holiday at our family beach house. Soon the sun would shine. Soon I would know what I was fighting. Soon the cancer would be gone.

The days dragged by. Late afternoon into evening was the worst. My illness was always on my mind. I tried to distract myself by watching TV or reading, but nothing could silence the terrifying thoughts of what the tumour was doing to my body. Knowing that I had more waiting to contend with meant more anguish and distress. Sleep was elusive. I was unable to stop my mind from playing games with me and going to scary places that I did not like. I was lucky to have four or five hours of sleep each night. I could not take this much longer.

At work, during my breaks, I almost wore a path in the carpet walking from my desk down the hallway to Systems, to unload all my fears on Ben and his colleagues. They always made me laugh and smile with their jokes and clowning around. Ben set up an old computer in the office among his colleagues and I became an honorary workmate in the Systems office. One day, while I was in Systems, Ben gave me his old laptop from home. He had loaded it with all his movies and music. The laptop became my new best friend and bedmate. That night, I replaced the spare pillows on my bed next to me with the laptop and at last reality faded. I was soon lost in whatever pulse-pounding thriller or love story was unfolding on the screen. I no longer watched the clock. Sometime between 2:00 or 3:00 each morning I would drift off to sleep. I woke up when the alarm went off. How many hours I slept was irrelevant. That I eventually fell asleep was all that mattered.

The tumour was turning into quite an opponent. I felt like I was in a boxing ring. By my reckoning, the tumour had won the first round. Waikato Hospital was unable to determine its pedigree and it was able to continue living in my arm. I felt that it was laughing at me, bouncing around my radius in victory.

It was the end of January and still no test results. The lack of information from the hospital was driving me crazy. I had to talk to my doctor. I decided to catch him after rounds and forced myself to go back to Waikato Hospital and wait in Ward 6 where I had recuperated from the biopsy operations. I needed to know if Auckland Hospital had reported on the last biopsy and when I could expect to hear the results. He told me that Auckland Hospital could not figure out what kind of tumour it was and had sent the specimen to the Mayo Clinic in Rochester, Minnesota, U.S.A. The results should be back by the end of February. More time to let my mind play horrid games!

I wished then that I had accompanied my tumour specimen to America. All I could think of was the interminable wait that I faced. I had this sodding tumour in my arm having a merry old time with absolute freedom to do what it wanted. Knowing I had another four weeks of thinking the worst about all the horrible things the tumour could be doing added to a growing sense of anger and frustration. The worst was feeling powerless. I felt stranded. I wanted someone to put me into an induced coma. I did not want to go through each day waiting for a call. I hated it when people asked, "How did you break your arm?" especially when shopping. All the attendants would ask this question because in the normal world there would usually be an interesting story associated with breaking an arm. If I said swimming, they would give me this uncomprehending look and I had no desire to give them a detailed account. I just gave them a very bored look and with a yawn in my voice I replied, "It is too boring to talk about." Further questioning rarely followed.

Welcome Diversion

A few days later, I had a date with a fellow (let's call him David) I met on a sports dating website. He was a welcome diversion. David lived in Thames and I agreed to drive over and meet him for coffee. Our conversation consisted of a seemingly endless series of questions about his participation in multisport events. The best thing about multisport is how many different things you have in common with others sharing this passion. There was the exercise, equipment, accessories, supplements, diet, training plans and of course skin-tight Lycra—I was never short of a question for him.

Time went by and we were soon saying good-bye to each other. David said he would call me later on that afternoon. Always the optimist, I believed he would. It was a beautiful day; the summer sun was shining—to drive southwest back to Hamilton would be crazy. On my mind was a beautiful blue sea with a white sandy beach a few miles north. Our family holiday home at Rings Beach, where I have enjoyed many summer holidays, was more alluring on this beautiful day, much better than driving home.

I turned my car around and went through Thames again. Thames was a wild colonial mining and Kauri milling town during the gold rush of the late 1800s. The shops along the main road have kept their Victorian architecture. Once, there were a hundred hotels catering up to 20,000 people. Thames boasted more inhabitants than Auckland during that period. The last six hotels from that era remain operating today—all they need now are horses tied up outside to make a great postcard.

Leaving Thames behind, I drove up the coastline passing through sleepy towns. Some had only one shop. I love driving the coastal road from Thames to Coromandel. Pohutukawa trees arch over the road in places and brighten the beaches all along the coast. Pohutukawas are known as the New Zealand Christmas tree by virtue of their profusion of crimson flowers during December and January. As I drove through Tapu, halfway up the coast, I remembered making this trip as a small child and Mum stopping to fill the car with petrol at the local shop. This was also the last shop to sell ice cream until we arrived in Coromandel, an old gold mining town only thirty minutes away. But it was the longest thirty minutes in creation when you are a child longing for the next rest stop. The winding coastal road of the Coromandel Peninsula held memories of sitting in the back seat of Mum and Dad's car eating lollies, ice cream, or ice-blocks with Allan and Gael in the summer. I vividly recalled eagerly watching for the house with a picture of Popeye in the window.

The familiar smell of seaweed rotting on the beaches drifted through my window making me smile as I looked out over the sparkling blue sea marked with people fishing from their dinghies. Leaving the coast road for the inland hills, I had to slow down for sheep crossing. There was always some animal to watch out for along this stretch. Nowhere else in New Zealand have I had to stop so frequently for sheep, geese and cattle. My trip to the family beach house was always interesting.

The drive to Rings Beach was beautiful. Navigating the sharp, twisty highway kept my attention on the road and off the lingering fears about my health. I was hoping I might get a phone call from David to meet up for a beer later that evening.

An hour and a half later I arrived at our family beach house. As I opened my car door, the smell of the salt air and fresh breeze was invigorating. The sound of the waves crashing on the beach enticed me across the road to the sand dune path. Many years ago two old logs were placed on this wide v-shaped pathway. The logs served as giant steps to the beach, and although now slowly rotting, they are still doing their job. Walking along the beach relaxed me. All of my fears flew away with the wind, as it blew into my face and through my long brown hair. The eastern end of this enchanting little beach has rocks to fish from and mussels to harvest. A creek to the west that I swam in as a toddler still holds such a special place in my

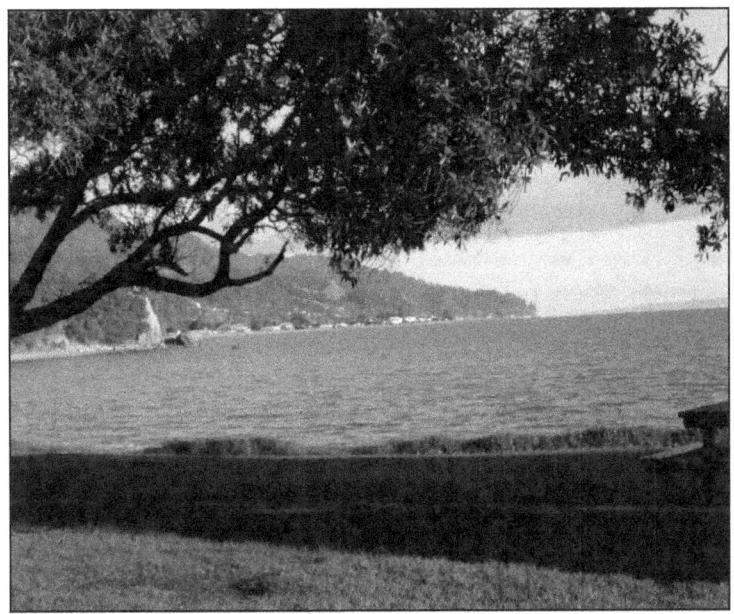

Driving along the Coromandel Peninsula

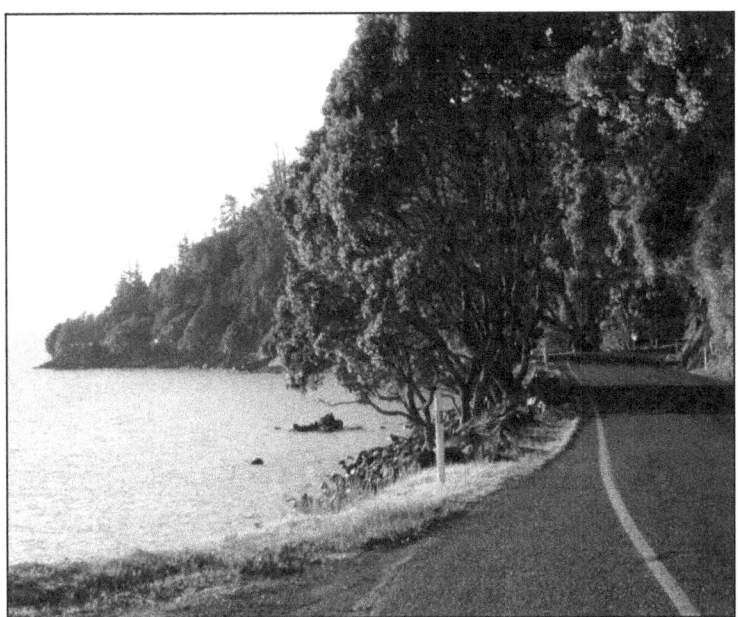

Driving along the Coromandel Peninsula

heart. Growing up here provided countless adventures as a child, a teenager and now as an adult.

Rings Beach was where I escaped for holidays and for rest and relaxation, as well as to recharge my tired body. Now it offered welcome relief from the constant buzz of what ifs and fear of the unknown.

I loved to meet up with all the local families I had grown up with, to catch up on their news and enjoy their comradeship over a drink or two.

Rings Beach has thirty or forty summer houses and everyone there knows everyone else. The beach has a few homes with converted garages or sheds ingeniously disguised as bars. One of them has a sign on the garage door "Always Open," with hats from all around the world hanging from the beams. While another bar has a Pirate theme. In one corner of the bar there is an old chest with jewellery falling over the sides among other fake treasure. John's bar is one of the originals on the beach and is like a museum with artefacts dating from his childhood. The

Dane's bar has a majestic view of the beach. From their elevated section you can watch the sun set drinking snaps and eating Danish delicacies. Most of the places have a downstairs fridge that is always full of refreshments.

At a beach gathering one year, after a few drinks, some residents of the beach bestowed upon John the title of Honorary Mayor of Rings Beach. Years later at another gathering, some residents thought it only fitting, in celebration of The Lord of the Rings trilogy winning so many Oscars, that Rings Beach crown an "Honorary Lord."

Walking back up the path, over the sand dunes then across the road, I climbed the stairs of our family's two story house. I walked to the kitchen, opened the cupboard, and lifted out one of Allan's bottles of red wine. I made a mental note to myself to replace it, and then took the bottle and a glass out onto the balcony to stare at the beautiful blue sea. I looked out over the large expanse of the Pacific

Ocean encircling the mainland and glistening in the afternoon sun. To the west lies the remainder of the Coromandel Peninsula. To the north and east are the Islands: the beautiful Great Barrier, then a short jump east to Cuvier, then Great Mercury. In the distance, the Red Mercury Islands, looking like one of the giant Easter Island statues lying down, showing the outline of a sleeping face and body. Sitting on the balcony sipping my red wine, captivated by the mesmerizing views, I manage to escape reality for a little while. It was nearing the end of the day as I watched the sun setting to the west of the hills of Coromandel. I had received no call from David, which upset me in a stupid way. I wish I had not been so optimistic. It would have saved me a lot of disappointment. My imagination was starting to drift into gloomy thoughts, which like the sky were getting darker by the hour. It was time I thought about heading home.

As I was slowly taking things to my car, Jane, a neighbour, came over and called, "Hey Barbs, do you want to come over for dinner? Mike and I have some friends here and you are welcome to join us."

Fighting to hold the tears back, I told her I was too miserable for company and didn't want to spoil her family time with my gloom. Seeing that I was upset she didn't push me.

"Hey, that's okay Barbs, but if you change your mind come on over for a drink."

"Okay Jane, thanks heaps."

I did not go over to Jane and Mike's for a drink—my mind was just in a bad place. Driving home in the dark, I turned the radio up loud and listened to Radio Hauraki. This helped to knock some of the dark thoughts out of my head. The trip back to Hamilton took its usual three and a half hours and I was glad to be doing something that kept my mind on "now." All the way home I listened to classic soft rock. I sang to the odd favourite song, but if a sad song came on the radio, I changed the station in search of something uplifting.

Things were just getting worse for me. How could I have had such continuously bad news month after month? At the end of January,

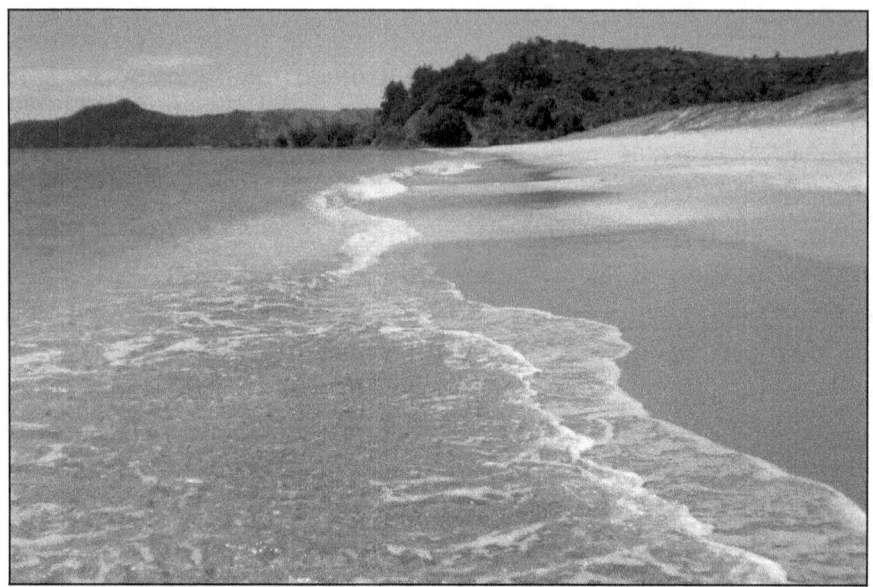

Rings Beach, Coromandel Peninsula

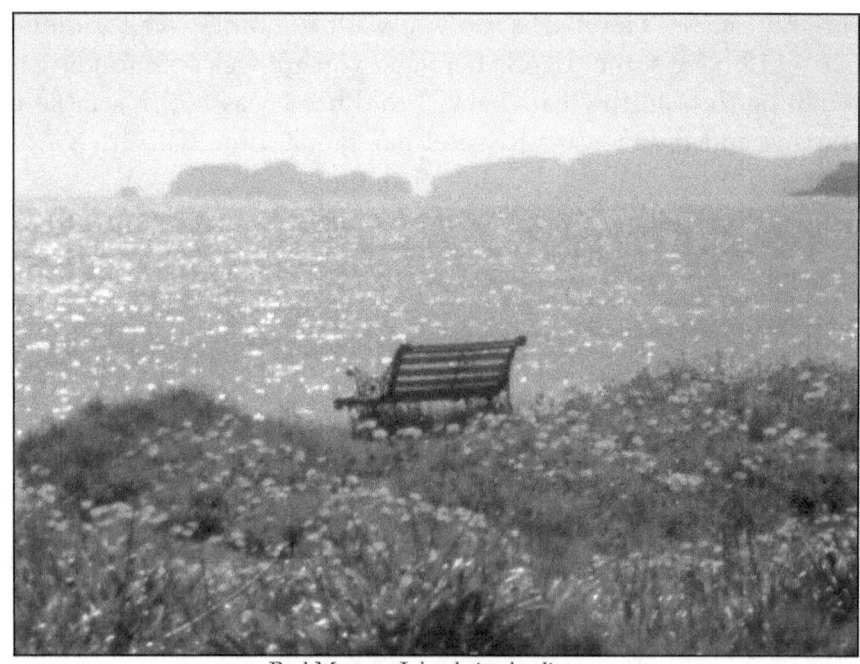

Red Mercury Islands in the distance

Grandma died. I could not believe that 2007 could start so terribly. February 7th, the day of my grandmother's funeral, I was waiting in Waikato Hospital on Ward 6 for the orderlies to arrive with a wheelchair and the long trip downstairs for an MRI.

I missed the funeral. As bad as it sounds, I mentally could not cope with it. It did not sit well with me when my mind kept creeping to the possibility of my own death.

A week later, my MRI scan showed the tumour had not changed in size, shape, or form. At first, I was ecstatic and then puzzled. Even the doctors could not believe it did not change its size. The doctors and I thought that tumours were always growing. I wondered if the rheumatoid arthritis medicine was having any impact on slowing the growth of this tumour. I googled my arthritis medicines and struggled to find support for my vague idea that these drugs might slow a tumour's growth. I figured whatever it was that was keeping this tumour small, it was fantastic.

The month of February was difficult for many reasons: David ceased all communication after the occasional brief call (cancer is a scary thing for friends and lovers to consider—it sure sorts out the friends worth keeping); Grandma died; and there were endless days of waiting for a call from my doctor. I had no control of the situation. All of this non-action made me wonder if the tumour in my arm was metastasizing. Worry kept on gnawing away in the back of my mind. Sometimes I would briefly forget my "death sentence," and then it would flood back. I hated every second of it.

On February 20, I finally received a call from my orthopaedic surgeon, Dr Hardy. I was at work, so I

walked away from my desk and down the hallway to where the reception was good. I rested my elbows on the windowsill as I looked out across the car park to the trees along the riverbank. I knew this was the call I had been waiting for.

He quite simply said, "I know you will appreciate being told now instead of waiting to come in and see me, as is the usual practice. There is no easy way to say this, Barbara, but you have a

Chondroblastic Osteosarcoma."

"What?" Thinking—that is quite a wheelbarrow of a word. What does it mean?

"Is that the bad one?" He had told me about a few different kinds of tumours and I struggled to remember their names. We were, of course, all hoping for the benign one.

Dr Hardy said, "Ah, yeah. I'm so sorry."

Immediately I said, "Okay, can you please chop my arm off tomorrow?"

Cautiously he carried on, saying, "Well, an arm and a hand are quite useful. We might not need to amputate at this stage. An oncologist will call you tomorrow with a time to meet and go from there. Please call me if you have had no phone call by tomorrow."

Adamantly, again I said, "You can chop my arm off, honestly! I don't want this tumour to grow any more than it needs to."

Now that I knew what it was, I seriously did not want this tumour in me. As stupid as it sounded, I had this fanciful thought of going home to the farm, getting an axe and just chopping my arm off. This would surely eliminate a lot of waiting and worrying and time off work.

Dr Hardy said, "Just sit tight and let us deal with this problem step by step. Talk to the oncologist and we will go from there."

"Okay, thanks for calling. I will keep in touch."

I walked slowly back to my office with a sick feeling in the bottom of my gut. How dare the sun be shining! Who said those birds outside in the garden could chirp? There is nothing good to chirp about in my world. It should be raining with such horrible news. I knocked on Ruku's office door (she was another one of my managers) and I just stared at her.

Ruku just looked back at me. She knew what I was about to tell her and quietly said, "It was the call, wasn't it?"

"Yeah," saying it staunchly, not wanting to show any weakness.

Standing up, Ruku walked toward me and just put her arms around me in support, asserting, "You are going to get through this, Barb. Steve and the rest of our team here will support you through this and will keep your job on hold until we know more."

"Thanks heaps, that means a hell of a lot. Well, I better head home now and tell my family."

I packed up my desk in a blur and in a daze I drove home, thinking how crazy life was going to be from now on.

I was not looking forward telling my family the bad news. I was determined to be positive and tell them it was all going to be okay. I would have chemotherapy, surgery, radiotherapy—any damn therapy—whatever it took to kill this horrible disease, and before they knew it, I would be back at work and training like a loon again for Ironman.

Later on that night, lying in bed in the dark I was thinking, "Thank goodness for the Mayo Clinic in America." I really wished I could have flown over and thanked the doctor who found out what kind of tumour I had. I wanted to give her a big hug of appreciation. At last, this tumour is cornered! Its name is revealed. It is no longer an unknown parasite in my arm. I think I have won this round, in my secret "boxing match" between the tumour and me. I have it on the ropes. We have won a round each. I am calling the doctor at the Mayo Clinic "House" as I just love that television program. I wished there was some way of saying thank you to her. All I knew was that it was the Mayo clinic in Rochester, Minnesota. I just said a prayer of thanks and vowed, when all this nonsense was over, to ask for a copy of my medical records from Waikato Hospital, find out who the doctor was in the Mayo Clinic, and thank her.

Chemo A New Vocabulary

February 26, 2007. On this beautiful, sunny morning, a week before the Ironman race that I could no longer do, I finished off my work for the morning before having another consultation with my oncologist. All I remember from this meeting was the oncologist saying how nasty this tumour was and hearing the words, "The faster you start chemotherapy, the better."

From that point on, the conversation between Gael and the oncologist continued without me. I had asked Gael if she could accompany me for support and to be the one in charge. I knew I would not fully comprehend the information discussed and it would feel like a nightmare. I wanted to save my energy for the fight, not struggle to learn a new vocabulary, a whole new language of fear and pain. Gael would keep things in perspective for me and take charge of the situation, so I could try to relax and prepare myself for the fight of my life.

"Every three weeks you will receive chemotherapy as an inpatient. There will be three cycles of neoadjuvant Cisplatin/Doxorubicin treatment followed by surgery, then three additional cycles of Cisplatin/Doxorubicin chemotherapy. The possible side effects include tiredness, alopecia, infertility, gastrointestinal upset, and bone marrow suppression that makes you more prone to infections and bleeding. Also, renal toxicity, neurotoxicity, hearing loss and, rarely, an Adriamycin-induced irreversible cardiomyopathy."

Holy shit! There better be some good news. I was facing infertility, baldness, kidney and possibly heart disease, hearing loss and chemo-brain. Where was the good news?

The oncologist continued, "Cisplatin is very unpleasant chemotherapy, but very effective. Cisplatin is used in conjunction with Doxorubicin and Dexamethasone. Unfortunately, Cisplatin affects your kidneys. The degree of damage is variable, but it is just one of the known side effects. Chemotherapy will take three days for each cycle, depending on how your body copes, as you might need blood transfusions. I don't think we should delay chemotherapy a day longer. Would you be happy starting today?"

Shaking with disbelief that it was all happening so fast, I just stared at Gael, trying to get strength from her presence. The fear reflected in my face. My gut felt like it was dropping through the floor. The unexpected horror of the whole situation was flooding over me in waves of nausea.

"Yes. The sooner I get this over with, the sooner I can start training again." I was beginning to sound a bit one-tracked, I know. I had lived to train for Ironman for almost a year, and it was hard to turn my drive to train off.

"Let me ring Ward 25 and see if they have a bed free."

"Sure."

The phone call seemed to last all of five seconds. I thought I wanted the bed, then again, I wouldn't have minded waiting just a bit to get my head around things. I looked out the window. Scaffolding framed the view of another hospital wing, which was less than the width of a tennis court away. The concrete walls were grey and uninspiring. Paint peeled off of the wooden window frames, which seemed held together with ancient spider webs. What a horrible view to see each day, no sun, no life. My tumour is like a fat spider weaving its web around me and leading me into a dark world of illness and fear. The oncologist replaced the phone noisily.

"You are in luck. There is a free bed for you. Do you have any questions?"

"I went to a fertility clinic a few weeks ago and asked about protecting my ovaries. In order to preserve ovarian function to some extent, they mentioned an option of ovarian suppression using GNR antagonists like Cetrotide while I have chemotherapy." I had hoped to have a family one day. "What are your thoughts on this?" I couldn't believe the question came out so clearly. It was prompted by something I had read in Lance Armstrong's book. Gael's presence was also clearly rubbing off on me.

"Medical ovarian suppression might not prevent your eggs from being damaged by chemotherapy, but will suppress your periods and ovulation. Even if your ovaries are protected, pregnancy might not be safe for you if your kidneys or heart are damaged."

"Oh, so it's not really worth having this then?"

"Not really."

How quickly our dreams are shed.

The oncologist quickly signed all the forms required for chemotherapy, and handed them to me to read and countersign. Gael and I made our way up to Ward 25. The receptionist gave us directions to the lounge where we waited for a nurse. I read the consent form for chemotherapy, while Gael rang Mum and Dad. The consent form gave minute detail about which symptoms were caused by Cisplatin, Dexamethasone and Doxorubicin. I showed Gael afterwards and she said, "You have some of these now: difficulty sleeping, mood swings, hallucinations and dizziness."

"Yeah right, you are so funny." Seeing the humour in it, we both laughed. The tension slowly eased from me and I replaced self-pity with restraint.

The lounge we were directed to had a lovely, big sofa; a huge, old TV; and a bookcase with some donated books, including (interestingly, I thought) *The Complete Cellulite Diet.* Mmmm… just what the patients here needed. The room was huge and, unlike the oncologist's office, had a lovely view of the lake, surrounded by old oaks and gum trees. A path meandered around the lake and I knew it would be a great place to travel to in my mind when things got tough. Any time I was a patient here and well enough to come to this room, I knew I would.

Gael sat in an armchair reading a recent magazine. I had too much on my mind to read. I reflected on threes: three chemo drugs, three weekly intervals between cycles, three days of chemo each time. Triathlon's three disciplines: swimming, biking and running. Chemo's three disciplines: needles, drugs, vomiting. My mind went around in circles looking for patterns, making connections where there weren't any.

Forty minutes later, Mum and Dad arrived, carrying a bag with some jeans, t-shirts, pyjamas and books for three days. Any time I am in the hospital I wear my normal clothes. I don't want to be just a patient—I want to be Barb with all my quirks and eccentricities. I want to stay real and alive and as active as I can. I plan to keep to my routine as much as possible—apart from the swimming and cycling, which will obviously be impossible.

After I read the two full pages of all the things that chemo could do to me, all the possible nasty side effects, I figured if I came out of this unscathed it would be a miracle. Some of the words I could not pronounce. Some of the side effects were incredibly scary. I really did not understand what I was reading. It was all so frightening. I decided just to think, "Okay this sucks. It is all terrible. It is all bad. Okay, I get this." The words all blurred together. I was glad my sister Gael was with me at the consultation with my oncologist that morning. I knew I would be bombarded with information. I knew as soon as the oncologist explained things to me, it would go in one ear and out the other, but Gael would remember. Gael would tell me later in words I would understand, even though it was all ghastly. Part of me did not want to think or understand anything. I just wanted this cycle of chemo completed. One cycle down, five to go was on my mind. I wanted to strike out cycle one in a personal best time. Just like in any sport, going better, faster, smarter. This was my goal with chemo.

After I signed the consent forms, a nurse took my family and me to my room and I settled in. Once I was settled I told them it would be okay if they left, knowing no one likes being in a hospital. It is just no fun as a patient, or as a visitor, so I said to them with a big smile that I would be just fine. It was strange, but I just wanted to be on my own. I think the only person I wanted with me would have been a boyfriend, if I had had one. I did not want to put my family through the unpleasantness of chemo. It was scary enough for me and I did not want them to see me upset.

Infused Napalm

Chemo was just fluid going from a bottle into my body, what was so scary about that? I was more worried about the side effects. Because I am a strong willed person, I tried to fool my mind by being strong and staunch about everything.

I heard the medical staff bringing in the prep gear for the chemo. I was soon to have my first bout of chemotherapy—infused liquid napalm for the tumour. I don't know how beneficial visual imagery is when confronting cancer, but I took wicked comfort in imagining my tumour withering in pain, consumed in hellish flames. I would take no pity!

I wish I had some photos up on the wall from home: photos of our wonderful family beach house in the Coromandel and photos taken with Gael while in Fiji admiring beautiful sunsets, photos I could stare at and get lost in while thinking nice thoughts.

Before chemo starts, I am given saline fluid to protect my kidneys. I was lucky to be admitted that afternoon. The sooner this starts, the sooner I will be finished, and the sooner this tumour will be toast!

By six o'clock that evening the nurses had double-checked that I was Barbara Mockford, patient number DFF3560, corresponding with their paperwork and my armband. The nurses were garbed in their uniforms, gloves and aprons. It was quite daunting having four nurses dressed like astronauts checking and double-checking everything connected to my IV lines. The name of the first chemotherapeutic agent they gave me was Dexamethasone, followed by Doxorubicin and finally, Cisplatin. The most awful sedative, Methotrimeprazine (also known as Nozinan), was put in my line and made me woozy and sleepy—it was truly revolting.

They give this drug to apprehensive patients because it calms them as well as settling nausea. But, because my head was swimming, the effect on me was the opposite. Talk about edgy. I told myself to try and remember to add Methotrimeprazine to my "Do Not Use" list of medications. There is such vast array of drugs, all with their own weird side effects and all of them acting differently on different people. Sometimes it feels like hit or miss to get the right cocktail for each person. In this game of trial and error, my job was to learn what my body liked and what it rejected from the smorgasbord offered. That way I could guide the medical team in making this less difficult for me and for them.

I questioned the necessity of every single thing the doctors and nurses did to me from that point on, and then I'd question why a particular drug or procedure was used. The doctors were very patient and explained everything to me. Even though I didn't always like their answers or explanations, I just had to accept them and get through it. The sooner I finished cycle one of chemo meant one less cycle I had to endure.

Thinking positively while enduring the nightmare of chemo, I always looked forward to the completion of cycle six because I knew that was my end date. That was the finish line I was striving for even though it was months and months away. I kept asking the doctors questions, hoping to hear them say, "You'll be okay." That was all I wanted to hear, and no matter how I phrased the question, the answer I desired was always avoided. They told me they would love to be able to say, "You'll be okay," but they were unable to make promises they might not be able to keep. "Barbara Mockford, You Are Cured!" replaced the mantra, "You Are An Ironman!" and occupied my future thoughts for several months.

It is amazing how those little words could end up meaning so much to me here. I ended up just telling myself, "I am going to be okay!"

I decided to focus on positive outcomes. The chemo is going to kill the tumour. The docs will remove the dead cancer growth from my arm and things will be hunky dory. I can do this. There are a lot scarier things that can happen to me than a few bottles of liquid fire going into my veins making me feel sick for the next five months. After five months I will be back at work, back in the pool, and back on my bike and life will just carry on, no biggie. I no longer visualized the Ironman finish line—it had been replaced by a cancer finish line. When this journey is over I am going to PARTY HARD...

Cancer is just another adventure to get through, an adventure way easier than my Ironman training. There will be no cycling in the searing, hot sun or cold, biting, southerly wind and rain for six days a week. I will sleep in (which I really enjoy), wake up and feel a bit yuck, but keep on going till July. Cool. Looking back, my optimism seems half-hopeful, half-hopelessly naïve.

The next day (Cycle One, Day Two in the lingo) Steve, my manager from Fonterra, made a detour on his way to a basketball game and visited me for half an hour or so. He was relaxed, naturally sincere in his concern and cheered me up immensely. Whenever anyone came to see me, I always acted bright and happy. I never let them see me feeling down. I might have looked terrible with my hair in disarray, my poor face swollen and puffed from the chemo, but that was okay. As long as I stayed buoyant and happy, my visitors would feel comfortable and positive. We talked shop a while which helped distract me and bring a bit of normality back into my life. Just before Steve left he asked, "Is there anything you need Barbs?"

"Well, I have to drink heaps of water to protect my kidneys, so it would be lovely to have some nice flavoured water."

"Yeah, sure, no problem, I'll get Ben and some of the guys to come up tomorrow with the water."

"Steve, can you tell everyone why I'm not back at work and stuff and that it's cool for them to come and see me?"

"Sure. I'll go to each of their team meetings and let them know, tell them that you say 'Hi,' and mention that they're welcome to pop in. Well, I'd better head off to basketball. You take care, keep smiling and just ring me if you need anything."

The next day after considering breakfast (hospital food plus nausea—not a great combination) the lab people came in for my daily blood test. This was never easy, as my veins had shrunk from the dual horrors of illness and too many needles. The doctors came through on their rounds, Ben and the guys arrived with my water and a portable hard drive that had tons more movies and music on it—it was brilliant! Progress, plus some socialization and entertainment.

Those three days of chemo were awful. Needles, pain, nausea, pills, food, feeling like crap. I queried the gauge of every needle that they put into me, and I learned very quickly what those sizes meant—the smaller the number the bigger the needle and the greater the amount of pain I would endure.

I was discharged to go home on Thursday, February 29th. One cycle of chemo finished, done and dusted, only four more months and five cycles to go. Home to peace and quiet and my own bed. No more wakeup calls at 7:30 a.m. for hospital breakfast, blood tests and flushing of the IV lines.

It's Just The Chemo

Friday, March 2nd, I woke up feeling awful. My friend, Nobby, came round to my place for a coffee and looked after me for a couple of hours. Having his caring company was a gift and I wish he could have stayed all day, but of course he had to go back to work and then home to his family. He said I looked terrible and should go to the doctor, but I said it's just the chemo and that I would go to my room for a sleep later. He left after making sure I was comfortable and as okay as possible. By lunchtime, I was feeling weird and experiencing random pins and needles sensations. I crawled into bed to have a sleep.

A courier driver woke me up and I bolted to answer the door. Excited about the delivery of my expensive Rudy Project sunglasses (another Ironman toy) I immediately opened the box and promptly fainted. When I woke, I was shaking like crazy. I knew this was not normal so I rang oncology outpatient and they told me to get myself to the oncology ward fast. Thank goodness I lived only three kilometres from the hospital. I rang my neighbour, Tracey, as I didn't think I would make it to her place without fainting. She lived only a few meters across the driveway, but it was just crazy fainting and feeling like this. I never fainted or felt this bad and it did not make sense to me. Before I knew it, Tracey was assisting me into her car and helping me up to the chemo outpatient building.

My blood pressure was down to 90 over 60 and I was weak and shaking like crazy. I had pain in the lumbar region of my back like I've never experienced before, accompanied by intense pricks from phantom pins and needles travelling from my toes to my nose. To top things off, I was icy cold and felt like I had golf balls under my skin—adding to my pain. I remember asking for blankets and wondering if the coldness meant I was dying. I was too scared to ask, too scared to know. They finally stabilized me two hours later. I was terrified and had clearly frightened the medical team. I was close to being admitted to the High Dependency Unit, where the sickest people go. I felt so alone, even though my family was just a phone call away, they lived forty minutes from the hospital and I didn't want to frighten them. I knew my family would have been there in an instant, but I was determined to be staunch and brave like the Kiwi farm girl I was brought up to be.

I was traumatized from all the injections. The worst was the ABG (arterial blood gas) test. The needle went into the underside of my wrist and into my radial artery to test blood oxygen and pH levels. I was surrounded by three doctors and several nurses, all strangers. My flatmate, Mel, was with me, but this was not enough to console me. She really is an angel, don't get me wrong, and a cardiac nurse as well and so caring. But it's times like this when you would like your very best friend or a partner with you, someone to lean on and take on all of the responsibility, make all the decisions, so you can just lie there and heal yourself. Or just lie there feeling like crap, comforted by their assurances, "It's going be alright."

I rang my brother, Allan. Although he empathized with my having gone through this awful experience, he was in the middle of milking cows and couldn't just stop and drive in. I realized by the time he arrived I would have settled down or fallen asleep anyway. I told him, "It's okay." Talking to Allan eased a certain amount of anxiety, as did a chat with Mum. I downplayed my situation so they wouldn't worry about me. Although my family was reasonably close geographically, they all lived too far away to be able to just pop in for thirty minutes or so. I knew my situation was better than other patients whose family lived much further from Waikato. I was fortunate.

My good friends, Nobby and Desiree, lived just a few miles away and I tried to ring them, but after the third or fourth try I gave up and admitted defeat. It was summer and I was sure they were out in the sun with their family and friends. I just lay in bed, staring out the window, watching the sky go dark blue with shades of pink, then into darkness. I was feeling lonely, watching the city lights switching on, then off, thinking of couples or families in those houses and slowly remembering what had occurred over the past three hours. I put my head down and silently cried the night away.

The next day the nurses told me I was dehydrated which was why my kidneys hurt like hell last night. It felt as if someone had taken a machete and sliced into each side of my ribs. The fault lies with the combining of my arthritis medication and the chemotherapy drugs. I was taken off all arthritis medication and I just hoped my arthritis remained suppressed throughout the coming cycles of chemo.

This had been the worst week of my life so far. Not only was I terribly sick because of the drug interactions, but my veins kept collapsing and the IV lines had to be replaced every few hours. I was a toxic pincushion, but that wasn't the worst part of my predicament. It was Ironman week. My illness meant I would not take part in the event I had been training for and I had optimistically settled on being a volunteer. I looked forward to hearing Mike Reilly say to every finisher, "You Are An Ironman!" even though I couldn't hear those words for myself. I wanted to hear my friends' names called, as one by one they finished the event for me.

I spent race day, Saturday, March 6, 2007, sitting in a hospital bed, texting all my friends to keep me updated on how Grant was doing. He was hoping to qualify for Kona (the Ironman World Championships) and this was to be his year. I missed watching the friends I made at the Ironman training camps in Taupo run over the finish line, especially Lauren, who I supported in the Rotorua Half Ironman. I knew so many people participating in the Ironman event. They were going to have the largest party ever in Taupo. Missing out hurt the most. I knew I should cry or emotionally unload because it wasn't healthy carrying it all inside. I couldn't say, "I have cancer." It didn't feel right saying it. To tell someone I have cancer and to see the raw emotion and the fear and then the pity on their face was just too much to handle. I am still trying to come to terms with it myself. Why cry over it? Crying wasn't going to make it all better. No magic wand was going to be waved over me to turn this into a bad dream and make it all go away. While I didn't think I would have any real release until my treatment was all over, I did know I would fight this parasite. I would come to terms with it behind a brave face and tell everybody I was going to be just fine.

I grew up on a farm, so I possess the outlook that if something bad happens, you fix it or kill it and move on. The worst part of this whole predicament was not being in control. Part of me wished I knew more about the armada of cocktails prescribed to kill this tumour so I could take a bigger role in the decision-making. I tell myself that when this is all over, a year or a few later, when I won't have to be staunch, be "bright, bubbly Barbs" to the world, when most of my fear has gone, I will go to my beach and find a rock and just quietly cry, washing away all the trauma I have gone through and cleansing myself of the demons that lurk in the background. I imagine it will be something really small that finally releases me. I will sit on those rocks all day, my eyes going red, eyelids puffing and tears washing down my face, while I listen to the waves crash on the rocks and appreciate what a beautiful but sometimes harsh world we live in.

Ironman day passes and so does my disappointment. Grant just missed out on Kona and is gutted. Lauren came in fourth to last and is elated—it's a funny old world.

I am all set to leave the hospital on Wednesday afternoon. One of the highlights of that week was a surprise picnic lunch organized by friends Kerry and Gareth. My hospital bed served as a picnic table. Cheese, grapes, ham, fresh bread rolls and the company of great friends—it was loads of fun and felt very healing. I think I ended up eating most of the food!

One of the bizarre things I found with chemo was that I got hungry and had the munchies quite a lot, usually occurring in the late afternoon and rolling into evening. Dexamethasone was the culprit. My meals at dinner were quite large considering how nauseated I was. The nausea peaked in the morning (considerably increasing my empathy for pregnant mothers). I would go from one extreme to the other and also had cravings. I went through a "cheese, crackers and dip" stage, making sure my cupboard was stocked with several different kinds of crackers, cheese, fruits and nuts. When I bought food, I did not care what it cost as long as it was of the highest quality and appealing to me. I couldn't settle for anything less than top quality—especially steak.

My commitment to eating well was confirmed one day while visiting Grant and his wife. He had just finished his triathlon training for the day and after a few drinks I told him I was cooking dinner. We went to the local market and bought the most expensive steaks, broccoli, potatoes and carrots—simple, healthy, tasty foods. Eating that steak was bliss. My whole outlook on food had changed. Instead of getting the usual everyday stuff, I went to the delicatessen section where all of the quality foods were kept. I refused to worry about the cost. I wanted quality, pleasure and satisfaction.

Cycle one was over and I was home again. Bliss. A week or so later, I found simply lying my head on my pillow hurt. My scalp was painful and I couldn't work it out. I had to stroke my hair and scalp gently to try to settle it. I decided to get a short haircut for a laugh. David, my stylist, asked, "What would you like Barb?"

"Oh something short, funky and fun."

"Why are you cutting your long, beautiful hair off? You have only just gotten the colour how you want it, and it's looking great!" David was horrified.

"Well, I have a sodding tumour in my arm and I'm having chemo, which is a real hoot. I will have no hair in a few weeks so thought I would have some fun with it while I still have some."

"Oh hell, that's no good about the tumour! But good to hear you're upbeat and positive about it all, not many folks would be this chirpy."

"Yeah, well, not much fun being around someone who is miserable, eh? And it just makes the other person feel uncomfortable. That would be just stupid I think."

"True."

While we were chatting away my hairstyle was taking shape. It looked so cool! I was excited about making such a big change. Shame it's probably not going to stay this way for long. My haircut cost $80. It was probably a waste of money, but I got $80 of great entertainment out of it and an idea for a new style when my hair grew back.

The third week in March my hair started falling out. At least now there were shorter strands of hair on the pillow instead of a foot or more from when it was long.

"Okay," I said to myself, "I am not going to let this fall out in dribs and drabs and have a patch-work scalp. I am getting it all off and over and done with!" Another trip to David at Kitzo, this time for a number one haircut. I rang Kitzo. The receptionist said it would be no problem and the cut would be free. Yeeha! How cool is that? With cap in hand I walked in to get my hair cut off. David was busy with a client, so another lovely lady came down to the reception area to take me through to the salon.

"Would you like to go somewhere private, Barbs?"

"Naah, it's okay, as long as the other clients are happy with me getting my head shaved."

"It won't be a problem, hon."

As my hair started falling off I became quite emotional. I came so close to tears while my head was being shaved. My hair had been beautiful and long and I had only just gotten the colour how I like it. I quickly pulled myself together and thought of the film *G.I. Jane*. It put a smile on my face. I just wish the same music was playing in the salon as when Demi Moore shaved her hair off. (I hate to think what was playing when Britney Spears did the same thing!) I thought, "I'm facing something almost, but not quite, the same as the *GI Jane* character." We both had to fight to win against the odds. I didn't want to know my odds because I didn't want to dwell on them. I just knew I was going into battle.

Wow, at the end of my haircut I had a round head, no embarrassing little bumps or flat bits, no nasty pimples or scars and I thought it looked quite cool. The one thing I noticed straight away was how cold it was and I was glad I had a hat to keep me warm.

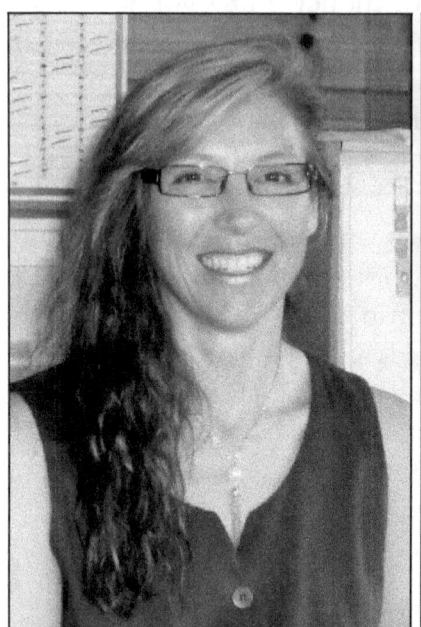

January 2007

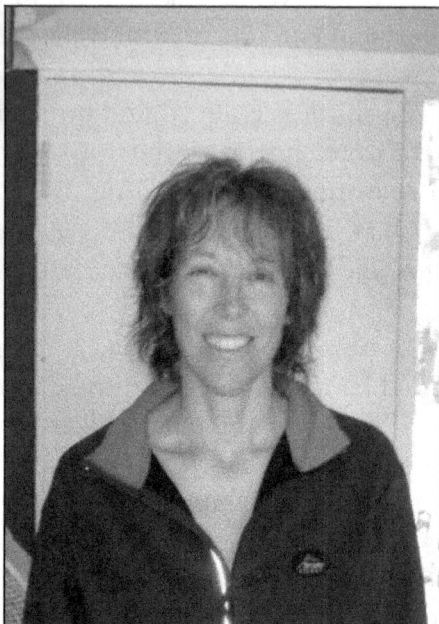

February 2007

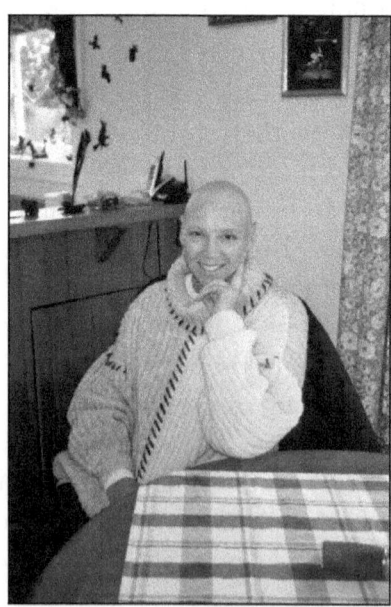

March 2007

March 2007 Cycle Two

Cycle two came round so fast. This time I was organized. I packed lots of DVDs and my internet-ready laptop. I was extra lucky to be put in a room designed for bone marrow transplant patients that had internet access. That was not the only wonderful thing in this room: there was a La-Z-Boy armchair, a little fridge, a TV with a video machine, beautiful curtains, and double-glazed windows with internal, automated blinds operated by remote. A five-star room! This was fantastic and I felt very spoiled!

Along with my other things, I brought an extra thick blanket. I got so cold all the time and hospitals just don't have real woollen blankets on the beds. I brought a bright crimson fake fur that was really cuddly. I also brought the treasured photos I wish I had up during cycle one. I had a photo of the beautiful beach I go to, a photo of Gael and me sitting on a beach at sunset in Fiji, another shot of a sunset in Fiji and an inspirational photo I was sent from a

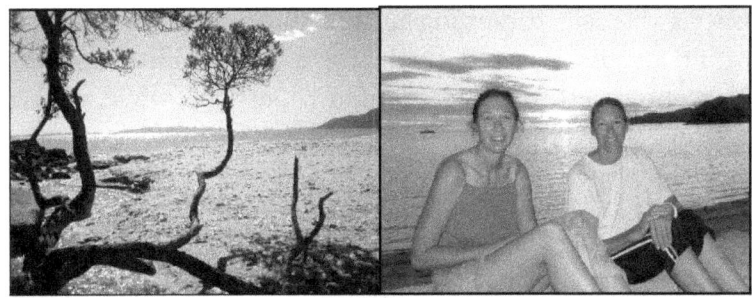

Wall Photos

friend taken while at Ironman 2007—yeah, the one I was meant to have done.

The guy in photo was running the marathon with a prosthetic leg. It was a modern carbon fibre running prosthetic. The photo inspired me and helped keep self-pity from setting in.

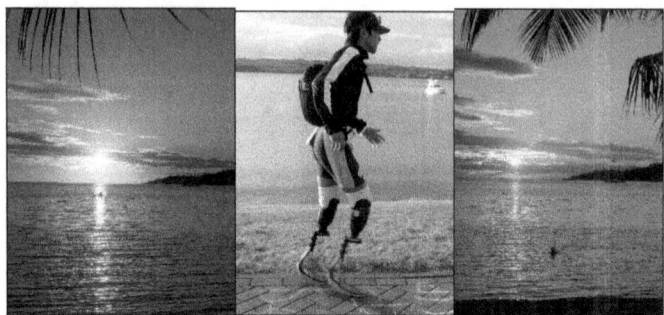

Wall Photos

The days that followed were hell. Whatever made me think this was going to be easy? I am just so blindly optimistic; sometimes it is one of my most annoying traits. I always think everything is going to be okay. My second cycle of chemo was pure savagery. It began on Day 1 when the nurses inadvertently gave me Nozinan again. I was so mad and anxious that I was again fighting that God-awful, sick, "out of it" feeling. Luckily, my friend Joy was there and she finally calmed me down.

I was so annoyed with myself that I didn't remember the drug issue from cycle one and failed to check what they were putting in my line. They call it chemo-brain. It felt like I had early onset Alzheimer's disease, forgetting all the important stuff, day by day. This would be the last and final time I would allow this revolting sedative to be given to me. I decided to ask the nurse the name of each and every drug going into my body. I might not know what they were, but to hear their names would give me back some sense of control.

Repetitive vomiting and nausea marked Day 2 of chemo, beginning at 6:30 Wednesday morning. I was given anti-nausea medication of all descriptions. I think I used their total arsenal of antiemetic drugs. It got so bad that by the afternoon the charge nurse decided I had been sick long enough and said she was getting a subcutaneous pump. This contraption allowed medication to be dribbled under my skin continuously over twenty-four hours. The evil bastard was inserted on Wednesday. I was already so sick and when I saw this damn needle and where the nurse was going to put it, I couldn't believe it. She aimed it at my chest just at the mid-line of a V-neck top, where it is all skinny and ribby. I requested a topical anaesthetic. The nurse said it's not that bad (basically she was not there to stuff around and meant business) and of course I thought, "Yeah, right, it is going to hurt like hell!"

That needle was the straw that broke the camel's back. I cried and cried—the whole business of where the needle had to go for starters, and then the realization that the skin on this part of the body is tough, which meant it was hard for the needle to go into. It wasn't soft like an arm and the needle seemed to take an age to go into my chest. This traumatized the hell out of me.

Half an hour afterwards, I was still upset about it and couldn't stop crying. I had to snap out of this and unload the ugliness of my day with someone. I flipped open my mobile and rang my brother, Allan.

Allan is the youngest in our family. However, I now think of him as my "big brother." Allan was returning for the night from a marlin fishing contest in the Bay of Islands. He'd been fishing several miles out to sea. He told me about his day and the crew he had on board. One was a local fisherman who took Allan and his mates to his favourite fishing grounds to catch the big one. Allan told me a long story about not catching anything that day and teasingly said he was sure the local fisherman was part of the "local Greenies" and made sure he didn't catch anything! This got me laughing. I could hear Allan's mates giving so-called "Greenie" heaps in the background and lots of laughter and the noise of the boat engine as they were motoring back. I so wished I could have been on that boat joining in all the fun. Allan and his mates' laughter cheered me up. I felt like I was taking part in something fun and joyful, not being stabbed and poked in my hospital bed.

Allan listened to my story of woe, all the horrible details, and said the things I needed to hear. Allan is a typical Kiwi bloke who says no more than strictly necessary. His phone calls are over in two minutes. His texts may contain only one letter, "k." Today, he knew what I needed and he delivered. He helped me escape my room of gloom and retreat to a place where everyone had a beer in their hand and told tall fishing tales.

All the warnings and lists of possible side effects had not prepared me for the repulsive smell of chemo drugs as they are excreted from skin and urine. This can last for days after the treatment. You're not told quite a few things—side effects vary widely—as obviously everyone is different. With some people, chemo does not cause hair loss. I wish I had been better prepared for the things that "might" happen, rather than experiencing them "blind." How great it would be if warned of the possibility of something bad happening and then finding you had escaped that one!

Odd things would happen and I ended up saying to myself, "Oh, okay. It's just another side effect. Marvellous." During my second cycle of chemo, I really noticed the smell—it's revolting and I felt so grimy and grubby. It was a metallic, acidic smell that just lingered on me. I wished I could go to a spa and have an all over cleansing body scrub to eliminate the smell. I decided that one day, when this was all over, I would spend an entire day at a Spa and have every skin cleansing option there was followed by all of the other luxurious indulgences.

My chemotherapy cycles ran every three weeks. By the time I was in the last week before the next cycle, the awful smell had pretty much gone from my body and I wanted at least another week to enjoy feeling clean. It was so frustrating. By the time I was feeling better and had some energy to really enjoy a nice long walk or go out and meet some friends without my constant companion, nausea, it was time for another cycle of chemo and that horrible smell once again ...

Unfortunately, the brief happiness after my phone call to Allan didn't last.

When they change bags of chemo, the nurses syringe a saline flush through the line to make sure it is clear for the next bag of drugs to go through. My line would not flush. I needed another needle. No matter how hard the nurse pushed down on the syringe (gently of course) it wouldn't flush. Chemo burns, it strips the vein walls of the protective layer covering the nerve endings so the most awful burning pain runs along the veins as the saline goes in. If the needle is not in the right place and the drugs enter the tissues rather than the vein, the tissues can rot and die. It is so important that IV lines are working and in the right place. I kept encouraging the nurse to save the line that was already in. At my request, he pushed harder and suddenly the saline rushed through. I almost leapt off my bed to the ceiling in excruciating pain. This set off my tears again. I told the nurse to set the pump connected to the bag on a slow rate so I could somehow get through this agony. I had to learn how these Ivac machines work so I could have some control and do it myself—set the flow rate and slowly increase it to the level the nurse wanted it to be.

Over the next hour, I slowly increased the flow rate to the required amount. It's so much easier inflicting small amounts of pain on yourself and being in control makes an enormous difference. After what I had gone through getting the last one put in, the prospect of getting a new IV line was unthinkable. I hated needles. It probably would have been better to have a new IV but there was a good chance that the drama of finding another vein would have been just as horrific. When the nurses did not have any success after the second attempt, they called in an anaesthetist—an expert in this area.

I don't think any nurse wanted to put an IV into my wrist as my tears added to the stress they felt just finding a vein. My wrists had to be put under hot, running water for twenty minutes so my cowardly veins would pop up. Even then, nurses struggled to find a suitable vein. The rest of the day I continued to feel sick and God-awful.

By 8:30 that night I had had enough of the nausea.

Screw this. I put my trainers on, grabbed a blanket, made a toga to go over my pyjamas and off I went, armed with a bottle of water. For the next hour, I marched up and down that ward and met a couple of true characters in their fifties. One of them was giving a nurse a good, humorous "curry up." There were so many different personalities on this ward.

Another bloke was wearing a Ministry of Works t-shirt and he looked like he would have a good story to tell over a beer. His story would have to wait—I was on a mission. I continued my walk, up and down, back and forth. By about 9:40 p.m., I figured I had covered at least a few kilometres and decided this would do. Surely the exercise would get the blood moving, the enzymes working, the muscles contracting, and get my system into some normality for the new day ahead. I had to have achieved something. It was training, in a limited sense, but I felt active again. If nothing else, I met two interesting codgers and got out of my room. I also exerted some control over the way I was feeling. In Ironman training, if I felt bad, I swam or ran or biked. Here, I walked and walked and walked.

Further compounding my horrible day was my oncologist telling me the next morning that I needed GCSF injections to increase my white blood cell count, since it had dropped terribly low as a result of my chemo.

White cells are the immune system's soldiers—they fight infection. I was told I needed to give myself an injection of GCSF into my stomach for the next seven days, and for another seven days after leaving the hospital following each cycle of chemo. You can imagine what I thought of that. Tackling it head on, I asked the nurse to show me how to do it while I was in the hospital and had her stand there while I did it. It was just totally foreign to me. These injections are the same ones diabetics have to do every day, the same size needle and syringes. The only good thing about doing it myself was I could put it into me as slowly as I liked. When the nurses did it, they did it fast and efficient and it stung like anything. When I took my time, it hardly stung at all. It took a lot to psych myself up to start the injection, but once the needle was in, it was no problem. The worst part was when I accidentally fumbled while supporting the syringe and it fell out of my hands leaving the needle still in my tummy. After doing that a few times, I never let it happen again. Lesson learned!

Unbeknownst to me, the next day my white and red cell blood counts were terribly low (neutropenia and anaemia) and were making my life crap. It meant my body wasn't strong enough to cope with the effects of the chemo. Chemo was supposed to be helping me; at the same time, it was making me very vulnerable to infection. A cold or flu could kill me. I found this out from my doctor during her morning visit. She told me if my blood counts weren't up later in the day, I would have to have a blood transfusion. My brain instantly leapt to "more injections" and I wanted to run at warp speed in the opposite direction. Refocusing on the big picture, I accepted the outcome. Thankfully, my counts later that day were up in the 90s and I got the four magic words, "You can go home," lifting my spirits to no end. I grabbed a taxi and headed home.

Progress

At home I emulated a cat—lying stretched out in the sun all afternoon, chatting away on MSN messenger to my mates and catching up on emails.

My tumour was definitely going down, I was sure it seemed less raised on my wrist. When my friend, Mandy, visited she tapped the tumour and told it, "Behave yourself and die!" This brought some appreciated comic relief. How funny to hear her sternly admonish my tumour to back off and die.

I thought I could feel progress. I had an appointment with my orthopaedic surgeon on April 5th for a consultation to discuss the extraction of the tumour, replacement of the diseased bone and fusion of my wrist. This appointment would surely be interesting.

Over the next few days, I slowly improved, but nausea was my constant companion.

My new routine went like this: wake up, walk in a dazed state to the kitchen, make a coffee, then go and sit in the lounge staring out my window at the garden and my neighbours. My neighbours were great. To the right of me was Elma, a nurse at Waikato Hospital who always allayed any crazy thought or concern I had. Looking out my window from my veranda, I could see Brad and Tracey's home. When Tracey was in her kitchen, she could see me having a coffee and we often gave each other a wave so she would know I was okay.

Most days, I would just hold my head in my hands all morning intermittently drinking my coffee. This might take two hours and two cups of coffee, or tea, depending how sick I felt. On a bad day, I started with tea and then progressed to coffee.

I didn't feel human till about lunchtime, then I would think about doing one piece of housework in the afternoon for the first week. This chore would be either washing, vacuuming, or just general house jobs. The following week was a bit easier to get through.

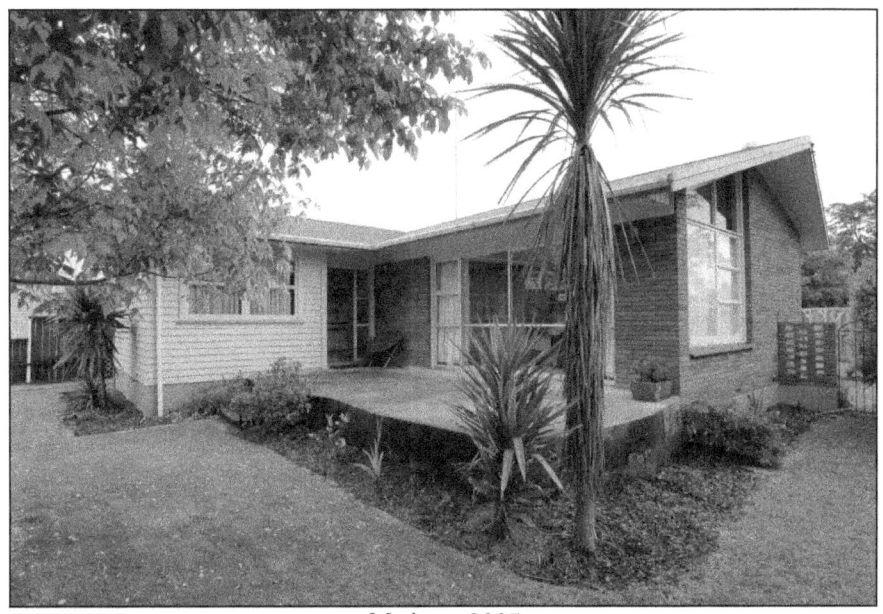

My house 2007

I was still struggling to come to grips with all the pills. I had a small pharmacy in a huge plastic box, including three different kinds of anti-nausea tablets: Ondansetron, Cyclizine and Domperidone. I found it so confusing in the beginning. When the district nurse came round to fill my subcutaneous pump (a huge syringe full of saline and Cyclizine) I got her to help me to draw up a schedule for taking my anti-nausea pills. It was important to take them regularly so I could feel almost normal. Chemo-related nausea is in part so horrible because it is always with you. I didn't think the feeling would go away until the chemo finished in July. If I heard of anyone feeling nauseated, I instantly felt empathy and heartfelt sorrow for him or her. The worst part was that vomiting didn't ease the sick feeling. When I vomited, I still felt like shit. Ordinarily, if I vomited I felt loads better afterwards and the nausea was forgotten. I never had this relief. The sickness remained 24/7 no matter what. I carried anti-nausea pills with me everywhere and tried to mentally remember when I had last taken them, not so easy with chemo-brain!

March 29th rolled around and I was only in day six of my release from the hospital and from the ghastly second cycle of chemo. Thinking of it still brings a tear to my eyes as I recall resigning myself once again to going back to the hospital. I felt just terrible, but what scared me the most was the torture of getting an IV put in. I put my bag together with my warm red blanket and my other treasures and rang for a taxi to the ED (Emergency Department). I was fast-tracked to see a doctor when I showed them the form I was given from Ward 25.

As usual, the young doctors struggled to find a vein big enough for the IV. It was put in a precarious place on the side of my arm and I just knew it was not going to last. The hellish part was when it took them four attempts to get a line into me, as well as three failed efforts to collect the huge syringe full of blood needed for testing.

Ward 25 was full, so I was admitted to Ward 4. As the orderly wheeled me there, I noticed immediately how quiet this ward was compared to 25. I knew my few days here would be relatively pleasant. I found one nurse who could put a needle in without it hurting, and that was a night nurse on this nice quiet end of the hospital. Knowing that the IV put in by the doctor in ED was not going to last, she put another one in at a different place. This nurse was the only one who got it right the first time and with no pain. I thought I was just dehydrated again, but I ended up neutropenic as well (I had a dangerously low white blood count). This was odd, as I'd felt quite good during the past two days.

The medical staff had so much difficulty accessing my veins and I experienced so much pain when the needles were inserted, that I wanted to have a hick, pic-line or portacath put in my chest to reduce the hassles with the IV lines. The portacath is like a socket they just plug the line into to download all the chemo. Once installed, this device would allow my doctors and nurses to take multiple injections from a single location. Not only is this a better and less painful experience for the patient, it also makes life easier for the medical staff. It seemed made for someone like me who is really scared of needles. The downside is that it is far more open to infection. My oncologist vehemently disapproved of the procedure for that very reason. Having a portal open to infection always present in a deep central vein was a recipe for disaster in someone with low white blood cell counts.

My low white cell count and anaemia had landed me in the hospital shortly after each chemo cycle. The chances of a hick or pic line becoming infected were probably high. The oncologist was just looking after me. It didn't stop me from being really pissed off at her. As my sister said, "If your oncologist was a bloke, you would not be so damn difficult!" And she is absolutely right—she knows me so well.

To cheer myself up, I remembered my bag of treasures and put my pictures up. This became a ritual every time I went to the hospital. Not only did it make me happy and provide a place to escape to and be inspired by, the nurses also loved the photos. Not one poor nurse left without a full description of each photo and the fact that I had missed out on Ironman! This will bug me for a long time. I have unfinished business with Mister Ironman.

The next day (Friday) I got progressively worse. My white cell count was low and I needed a blood transfusion. At 1:00 p.m. I was shifted up to the chemo ward where I was basically quarantined and could only eat specific food or packaged food. I requested rice and peas for dinner, because my mouth now had awful ulcers and my taste buds had gone haywire. These were the only foods that tasted like they should, so much food had lost its normal flavour, which was something I was getting used to. Ulcers in my mouth always occurred around day ten after the start of chemo.

I ended up drinking a lot of soup. The consistency of bread or products made out of flour felt awful in my mouth. I may as well have put a spoon of flour in my mouth—that is what bread, cakes, pasta or biscuits tasted like. After one bite there was great disappointment followed by spitting the food out and throwing away the remainder. What I missed most was munching on marmalade-layered toast or biscuits. When I figured out my dietary requirements, I made very nutritious vegetable soup each time I got home. I blended it and sprinkled corn and parsley on top before freezing for future meals.

Before they shifted me to Ward 25, I made a plan, as I just could not face the ghastly, boring, steamed rice and green peas I had ordered for lunch. So what if this was the only food that would not hurt while I ate. I remembered the smorgasbord of food in the hospital café—real food seemed like a damn fine idea to me. I told the nurses I was going for a walk and almost ran to the lift that would take me to where I would follow the infamous red floor of the Waikato Hospital then up another two floors in a lift to reach the café. I was still attached to my pole and line with fluid. I bought a huge packet of sushi—it felt like I had escaped from jail. It was so funny, but at the same time I quickly searched the area where the staff had their lunch in case any of them were from Ward 25. I raced back to my room, got there just in time and was halfway through my sushi, enjoying every second of it. God it tasted magnificent! It didn't sting the ulcers on my tongue or mouth and tasted divine! While I was happily eating my sushi, a nurse came in and gasped.

"What are you eating?!"

"Sushi, and it tastes great, the yummiest food I have found in weeks that doesn't taste like shit," I told her with a big smile on my face.

"You are not allowed to eat fish! You're neutropenic!"

"Goodness, what does that mean?"

"Your neutrophils are below 0.5." She saw the "What the hell does that mean?" look on my face. Sure, the medical terms had been explained to me, but I think that medical professionals forget that their words are a second language—one that doesn't mean anything when you are sick and tired, and tired of being sick. "It means that your white cells, the ones that fight infection in the body, are so low that any little bug could cause an overwhelming infection and kill you—the kind of little bugs that might be in your sushi."

"Oh." Not much the wiser, and determined to enjoy my meal, I thought I would ask her more about it later as she seemed a tad upset. When she left me, I decided to eat the rest of the sushi since I'd had half already. What the heck? I may as well eat the rest and enjoy it before the doctors arrived to shift me back to Ward 25.

I dreaded going up to Ward 25—it was so noisy. The background was always filled with the sounds of beeping machines administering chemo, intercom system chat and round the clock visitors. I think I am just used to a quiet house. I am so "Miss Boring" these days.

That Friday night in the room next door to me, a family was singing till 9:00 p.m. Okay, it was the patient's birthday, but how many songs do they have to sing; don't you just sing "Happy Birthday" and that's it? Not this party, there was song after song. I said to my nurse, "The singing stops at 9:00 p.m."

And he said, "Yup, I agree."

Sure enough, 9:00 p.m. rolled around and the singing stopped. I hope it wasn't the last birthday that family spent together. I was sick, and tired, and needed some rest. I did not feel apologetic for my irritation.

I escaped the need for a blood transfusion that week, and I was rapt. I was living quite precariously and would not have been too surprised if I needed at least one more over the next few months.

Oncology Nurses

I saw my orthopaedic surgeon at Waikato Hospital on Thursday, April 5th. He is a character who always has a cheeky smile on his face. He was still struggling with the fact that I had a tumour in my wrist, as it was so small. I don't think he would believe it if the Mayo Clinic in the States hadn't diagnosed it. The last MRI test results on the 7th of February showed that the cells were "non-aggressive," with no change in the size, shape or form of the tumour since the MRI of December 2006. Osteosarcoma is usually a very aggressive tumour. Perhaps my rheumatoid arthritis medication suppressed it. I sure hoped it did. I just clung with relief to the fact that the tumour was not behaving viciously.

The oncology nurses are truly amazing. Even though I was going through an awful time, the nurses were caring and skilled. I don't know how they do this job. The nurses did everything they possibly could to make my time here as pleasant as it could be. They got me ice-blocks whenever I wanted one. Sometimes I brought in my own food and ice-blocks. The patient kitchen stores all your favourite food if you bring it in. They let you make the ward as homey as you feel like making it. They are the most beautiful people you could wish to have at your side during this most awful time in your life.

The nurses are there during the embarrassing personal things you must go through, like measuring urine. They help you get through retched vomiting spells, replace the sheets on your bed two or three times in one day (after you vomit or sweat on the clean ones), put catheters in (that had to rate as another all-time bad experience), and expertly answer questions you never expected to ask. The relentless nature of cancer treatment and investigations makes even small hurts seem intolerable over time. The nurses helped me survive the indignity and discomforts of chemotherapy.

I was booked for another CT scan on the 23rd and an MRI on the

26th of April. I hoped these tests would confirm that the tumour cells were dead, as well as tell the surgeons what they needed to know for the operation in Auckland. The operation was scheduled for May 13th and there was only a small window of time to have the operation before my next cycle of chemo.

Life must also go on. I met another man on a dating website. He wrote lovely emails that lifted my spirits and took my mind off things. He made me feel special. He lived in Australia and we hadn't met yet. All of our contact was electronic—which made it more fun. I needed any kind of enjoyment just then.

A note from my diary at this time: "Tomorrow I start another round of chemo. I wish tomorrow was not tomorrow. Why couldn't tomorrow be 2008? I don't want tomorrow. I don't want it to be tomorrow. I wonder how many people are thinking the same as me? The barbaric torture I have to go through tomorrow shouldn't happen in this advanced society we live in."

Another round of chemo—it should only be three days, all going well. With me, lately, it never seems to go well. This round stretches to four days. The fourth day is spent watching my blood counts, which are always struggling to be in the normal zone and invariably just reaching their minimum upon departing the hospital.

They can put a man on the moon, but they can't put a needle in my vein till the third or fifth attempt.

Every first day of every chemo cycle is the same. Did I mention that chest skin is actually quite hard to get a needle into? We were down to the skin on my chest—every other site was scarred and useless. You just can't win in the world of chemo unless your veins pop out. Mine run away and hide at the mere mention of IVs. This made my life in chemo the pits. I pitied the poor nurses trying their hardest to make the experience less traumatic, but my patience was wearing thin.

The only time my veins would have been easy to put a needle in was when I was in Fiji a year earlier with Gael. I was healthier, and in the tropical heat, my veins stood out and flowed with life. A year before the chemo I was counting down the last ten days before getting on a plane for Fiji. Oh to be there now, away from chemotherapy where I waited for someone to put the IV line in after my sedative took effect, after holding my hands under the hottest water endurable to make the reluctant veins pop up.

The Claw

Twenty minutes before leaving for the hospital, I covered my wrists with Emla topical anaesthetic gel and bandages. Once again, with little enthusiasm, I packed my bag and took my sedative (the last two cycles were so traumatic that one of my doctors prescribed a sedative). I got into my silver MX5 and drove to the hospital for another three days of chemo. I timed it so that I arrived at the hospital just as the sedative started to kick in—how convenient living only three or four kilometres away.

At Ward 25 reception, I chatted with the nurses, put in a request for the five-star bone marrow replacement room and struck it lucky again. The receptionist was bright and bubbly and it was nice talking to her while she sorted out which room I was assigned to. Being a receptionist, I joked as I offered to do her job for a few hours so she could take a break. I often wondered if she and the many other hospital workers realized how important they were to patients so much in need of simple kindnesses and respect. The orderlies who shuffled me back and forth in my wheelchair always had a kind word and smile for me. These folks are an often underrated part of the team that makes or breaks a person's will to keep going.

Once in my room, I got out my photos and pinned them to the wall, smiling from the memories they inspired. I laid my warm crimson blanket on my bed—this made it homier and the nurses loved it too, so bright and happy. Each cycle of chemo I seemed to have different nurses and once again they asked about the photos and they all got the same stories, emphasizing how I missed out on Ironman and how this sport indirectly saved my life. I would not have taken any notice of the lump on my wrist, believing it was arthritis, if it weren't for the fracture sustained in the Half Ironman event. I will always be grateful to Ironman for uncovering my cancer before it was too advanced.

I have to say the first two days of my chemo went well. Despite being really scared about the pending IVs being put in, I was well-prepared. Amongst the treasures in my bag, I had Class 5 earmuffs from NZ Safety. They are industrial strength, useful here as Ward 25 is so damn noisy and I am a light sleeper. What I hated most was the relentless sound of my Ivac machine, as well as the machines for other patients continually beeping. So here I was, sedated up to my eyeballs with earmuffs on, waiting to be stabbed by the torturous IVs. In my relaxed and sensory-deprived state, I must have dozed off.

"Hello?"

"Hello?"

Why is someone shaking me awake? I was having the most relaxing sleep thanks to the sedative. The doctor had to shake me awake, as I couldn't hear him.

"Oh, hi!" Slightly embarrassed, I sat up to let him commence torture by a thousand needles. "Right, I want you to put one IV in my left hand and the other in the right. The one in the left will be for the saline potassium flush and the right for the chemo."

"Why ever do you want to do that?"

I explained, "This will prevent the agony of the potassium saline flush being put in the same IV line as the chemo. The chemo is really harsh and after the chemo, the potassium in the saline stings the hell out of my worn-out, raw nerves lining the wall of my veins."

Gee. I was starting to sound like a medical procedure manual. I had become quite assertive and I was now helping to choose how the cycles of chemo were going to go. I had decided to take as much control of each cycle as I possibly could. No longer would I just sit there and let things happen to me. If something could be done in a more pleasant or easier way, I requested it. The worst the medical staff could say was, "No." I also asked questions each time the nurses arrived with syringes to be put into my line, "What is this drug?" And, "Why is it being given?" The fear of it being Nozinan was always at the forefront of my mind. There was no way I wanted that medication again. It might be wonderful for other people—it wasn't for me.

Thankfully, the doctor went along with my request. The IVs in each hand went in well, so there was minimal chance of them blocking or leaking into the skin tissue (which has happened two or three times and it hurt like hell for ages). Maybe this cycle would be a breeze.

Day three was ghastly—so much for thinking this cycle was going to run smoothly. I was sick all day. Later, I found out that the shutter had been left closed on my subcutaneous pump (the pump that continuously shoots anti-nausea medication under the skin via a needle in my chest). I think the night nurse was a trainee; the poor thing was devastated when she realized later that she had caused me to feel so terrible. I told her in an upbeat voice that it was okay and not to worry about it. I was sick all day, but tried to take it in stride and not make her feel too bad. But by God, I won't forget this next time! It's another thing to remember for cycle number four in June.

On discharge day, I was so excited! Each cycle was different— new things went wrong, new things went well, but the wrongs somehow seemed to overshadow the rights.

Almost sprinting out the door with all my paperwork and prescriptions, I jumped in my car and savoured being happy again. If I was lucky, I wouldn't be back for another three weeks. I drove to the chemist and ended up paying $180.00 for four different kinds of anti-nausea medicine, saline, and other bits and bobs. Unreal. So much for our "free" public health system! Thank goodness I had medical insurance.

The next few days at home, I felt like I was walking on a thin ice shelf, waiting for it to collapse. In my mind, going back to the hospital was a thing to greatly fear. So many things could go wrong, a creatinine build-up from kidney damage, or neutropenia and anaemia from bone marrow suppression. It felt like doom surrounded me. I thought that if I could get past day six out of the hospital it would be fantastic.

On Wednesday, I went to "Feel Good, Look Good," a program run by the Cancer Society. It was brilliant. Up until that day, I had no interest in putting make-up on. I would wake-up, look at myself in the mirror and think, "What an ugly sight!" I didn't feel female or male, just generic. I felt blah and sexless and it seemed pointless to make an effort to look nice since I felt like shit most of the time. I would go everywhere barefaced, wearing a cap or woolly hat. I'd bought a lovely wig, but after an hour or so it irritated my scalp and I had to take it off. I think the longest I wore it was two hours. "Feel Good, Look Good" brought back my confidence and feelings of femininity. I was so grateful.

After the make-up and pampering session, I noticed my nose was sniffly, and I thought, "Oh God, where will this go?" By Thursday night I was feeling dreadful and had chills. I woke up Friday, April 20, with a temperature of 38.5°C (101.3°F), and thought, "Crap!" I took some paracetamol and drank lots of water and the fever went down half an hour later. I put myself back to bed and slept. I did this a couple of times throughout the day, staying in bed, desperately trying to fix myself to avoid going to the hospital which always meant pain and needles. I am one tenacious, stubborn female and wanted to cure myself. By 4:00 that afternoon, the fever peaked again at 38.5°C and I reluctantly gave in, knowing more needles and IV lines lay ahead of me. I packed my bag, rang myself a taxi and half an hour later I was once again in the hospital. I had managed to stay home seven days.

I was too sick to waste time applying Emla gel and was not sure where they would put the IV as all my visible veins were stuffed. I also forgot to take the sedative this time, so I just had to try and tough it out. Sure enough, they struggled to find a vein. After the third attempt, they found a vein on the outside edge of my arm. I knew this was not going to last until the next evening. From the Emergency Department, I was transferred to Ward 25. Once in my room I got out of bed, opened my bag, put my red blanket on my bed, collected my pictures, wobbled over to the wall with my Ivac machine, put the photos up and smiled at them. The IV on the side of my arm ended up failing the next day. It was blocking the whole time in the Ivac machine and stung like hell when they flushed it because it was leaking into skin tissue. To top things off, I had painful ulcers in the back of my mouth and under my tongue, as well as on my palate and up both sides of my mouth. I struggled to eat. I couldn't eat anything with flour in it—everything tasted odd.

That night, there was a God-awful moan that turned into a blood-curdling, screaming yell from somewhere down the corridor. I thought someone's relative had died or they were being tortured or something—the noise went on and on for five to ten minutes. Later, my nurse came in to check my observations.

"Who was killing that bloke down the hall?" I asked, irritated.

"Oh, he fell over in the bathroom, the poor guy. I am just going to check your OBS. How are you feeling today?"

"I am tired and I want a strawberry milkshake and muesli with fruit and nuts for breakfast."

"You know you're not allowed those foods when you are neutropenic, but I love your humour," she said with a laugh.

The guy down the hall gave a repeat performance that evening, slipping in the bathroom then screaming in pain. In my haste to get into the hospital this time, I had forgotten my earmuffs. I needed my earmuffs. I needed my Emla gel. I needed my mum. And I needed to go home.

The next day I had a blood transfusion that took a whole day. I don't like blood transfusions as they hurt a bit from the speed that the machine pumps the blood. I always put in a request for "teenage blood" as a standing joke. If you have a choice, why not get the youngest, most energetic, hormone-loaded blood?

I finally escaped the hospital. Oh what a celebration! I felt like hitting the town and going mad with my MasterCard for some retail therapy and loads of fun. But, nope, the poor credit card will be buying two boring tires and some petrol. It will seriously need to be cleared next payday.

I treated myself to a trip to Rotorua to watch my friend, Lauren, finish the Rotorua marathon. I planned to support and cheer her on all day, as I had hoped to do for the Ironman before cancer spoiled my plans. It promised to be a blast. I went out there with my pink pom-poms, cheering her on, and, of course, every handsome bloke with good legs who happened to cross my path!

My operation was scheduled for the 13th of May. The chemo-weakened tumour was to be cut out and my diseased forearm bone replaced with the fibula from my leg. My new wrist would then be fused with steel and screws. I already had a new nickname, "The Claw." My mate Kerry called me this—what a hoot! I thought it was appropriate and liked it straight away. When I do the Ironman, I will be putting this name somewhere on my race number tag or t-shirt.

It's a big operation—scheduled for five and a half hours. I will be in Manukau Super Clinic for at least ten days. I will check in on the 12th to get prepped and tested a day before the operation. Mum makes plans to stay at a nearby hotel for a couple of days and I demanded that my brother Allan be with me after the operation. He is my leaning post when life gets ugly.

Meantime, it is getting wintery and I have put a new flue in my fireplace. It really sucks because it cost five hundred dollars and looks no different than the old one. At least it shouldn't leak smoke and my house will be toasty warm and pleasant again. Small things make me happy these days. I don't know if this is normal or just the chemo having an effect on my brain.

Don't Let Me Down

Isn't it weird that when something major happens in your life you see it on TV? Sometimes, if you're having an affair, a fight with your best buddy, or you're in a bad relationship, your situation crops up coincidentally in a program on TV. You get to see your own story told and acted out by people you don't know. I wonder what all this means? A coincidence? Karma? I just watched an episode of *Bones* on TV. A deceased victim on the show had sarcoma in his groin and hip (they found his bones). Wednesday, on *CSI*, I heard the word "osteosarcoma" and they mentioned the immune system. I had this crazy idea that I might learn one tiny thing on the programs that might help me. It feels really stupid, and I realize I am grasping onto anything that I can to help, no matter how remote it is to my situation. It's part of taking back control, I think.

I am finally feeling a bit better. God, I feel like pinching myself to prove I'm not dreaming! Then I get chemo again and the brief feeling of well-being disappears.

My March stint in the hospital was truly horrible. I ended up with a sub-cut pump and demanded Emla gel before anyone put another needle into my chest—but the Emla only stops a portion of the pain, and the pump only kills a bit of the nausea, and tears are always shed afterwards. Each time I enter the hospital, I wonder if I will make it past day six and leave the hospital. My brief break after each blast of chemo always ends with a lonely, impersonal taxi ride back to the hospital.

My body does not take chemo well. Does anyone sail though chemo? I know I am not alone and that offers some consolation. In a nutshell, my immune system must be saying, "What the hell are you doing to me?!" The treatment knocks me for a loop and it gets rougher and harder to crawl back to some semblance of "normal" after each cycle. I feel myself getting weaker and weaker no matter what I do. Once again, I realize the logical and sensible reasoning my oncologist had for not letting me have a port. I still resent the necessity of pricking me with needle upon needle, though, as a result of not getting a central line. Logical thought is not always the order of the day when dealing with cancer.

My oncologist gave me the maximum dosage of chemotherapy each time. She said she did not change or lessen the dosage despite my reactions because she wanted the drugs to produce the desired result. I appreciated this. There is no point tiptoeing around this osteosarcoma critter; you don't want it to stay strong enough to turn round and bite you. That being said, my poor immune system suffered a knock the first time, a double knock the second time and on the third time, it struggled to fight back.

My diary again: "It is like I am stuck in the most never-ending nightmare and can't wake up. It feels like I'm diving ten meters underwater with the greatest pressure weighing on my body and I'm slowly fighting to get to the surface to see the sun shining, but I never ever reach there. I am weighted down, perpetually struggling and fighting and kicking like hell for the surface. The horrible thing is, I will be living this nightmare for another three months and three cycles before reaching the surface, the sunshine and fresh air. Can I survive and break through to the surface?"

I stay up the night before I check in for surgery to watch Team NZ race Luna Rosa in the America's Cup. This is the first race I have stayed up for—it is quite important as the next one is against the defender, Oracle. It will be a good race, I just hope the wind is more than ten knots and there is plenty of action, and Team New Zealand gets some really good windward lifts. I realize I am also rooting for my new home team: my team of doctors, technicians and nurses.

My appointment with Dr Gary French is at 10:00 a.m., May 8, and is a three-hour consultation. Wow, three hours!

The surgeon sounded really nice on the phone. He told me there is still a chance when they open me up that they may need to amputate my arm.

I said, "Hey, go for it! I want live for another fifty years, not days or months."

He said, "Yeah, we need to discuss this when you're up here on Tuesday."

I was really interested in hearing how they would perform this operation. A team has been looking at my MRI scans, preparing themselves for the operation and planning their strategy. As long as I can cycle 180 kilometres and walk 42 kilometres after the operation, they may cut and paste where they like. I saw them as my hospital team rallying to help me keep Ironman in my sights. Waking up from the anaesthetic on the 14th to see whether I still have a hand or not was something I didn't want to think about, but the possibility of losing my hand was real and in the back of my mind.

Gael travelled with me to see Dr French and review all my medical checks. I had more X-rays of my arm, an ECG and all the normal things like blood pressure measurement. Before I knew it, I was called from the waiting room to see the doctor. I usually let Gael do most of the talking with the doctors, especially the ones I felt nervous around. However, I liked Dr French straight away and we both agreed I would address him as Gary. He chatted with me about things that would happen in a way I was able to easily understand. He didn't make it sound complicated and had such a great, positive personality that I was able to trust him from the start. A doctor's "bedside manner" should never be underrated. I believe it seriously contributes to the outcome of treatment, be it positive or negative.

Gary said, "I will be removing your tumour and will use the fibula bone from your leg to replace the radius bone that will be removed. I will need to take out your carpals—the little hand bones—as well. There is a strong chance I may need to amputate your arm above the elbow, halfway up your humerus, depending on how much of the radius is affected by the cancer. You need to be prepared for this possibility."

"That's okay. As long as you can keep me alive, you just do what you would do if it was your own arm. If you take the bone from my fibula, will I be ever able to walk 42 kilometres and cycle 180 kilometres?"

"Yup—but you won't be able to run it."

"No problem." I thought of my picture of the man finishing Ironman on artificial legs. I could walk the Ironman marathon with arthritis and a missing fibula. I needed to keep the Ironman dream alive—in my mind as well as my surgeon's. Finishing the Ironman is a goal, so big it seems unreal, that keeps me striving onwards and reminds the surgical team that I have dreams beyond the operating theatre.

Gary would also be fusing my wrist, so a titanium rod would be inserted inside my fibula, with a plate at each end screwed into the fibula and remaining radius at the elbow. At the end where the fingers are, the plate would hold the fibula in place with two screws angled down each side of a metacarpal joint followed through with two in the remaining fibula to keep things strong. I was beginning to feel like the bionic woman without all the benefits, but I will be alive.

I left with Gael in a very positive spirit and feeling that at last something good was about to happen. My horrible tumour would be removed soon. No longer would the cancerous mass of cells be part of my body! I had a fantastic surgeon in charge of my remodel and no more chemo for three or four weeks. All this "good news" made me feel like having a huge party. I felt good again!

I counted on my CT scan to show a clean set of lungs, heart, kidneys, stomach and liver. The last two were clear, but I requested this CT for my own reassurance. The surgeons can have the MRI, but the CT is for me.

My body didn't let me down. The scans were clear and hopeful.

Surgery

May 13, 2007. My day under the knife had arrived and as I was being wheeled to surgery I was thrilled to see Gary and Mary. Mary is a close friend of mine—a nurse who works in pre-op prepping patients for surgery. It was lovely having her there to stay by my side and talk me through all the strange things that happened. My anaesthetist tried to put an IV in my arm. I didn't say anything to him about my veins because anaesthetists are gods when it comes to putting lines in—they are just brilliant. Not surprising to me, but enormously shocking to him, the anaesthetist failed on his first attempt. I found it quite funny. He had to put up with "second time lucky." How disappointing to be human!

However I came out of this operation, I would be better off. The tumour in my radius would be gone—obliterated, destroyed. There was no evidence that it had spread yet; let's get rid of it before it decided to. I would be free of the constant worry that it was on the move, spreading like a sneaky, invading army.

Next thing I knew, I was awake in recovery crunching an ice-block and chatting to someone across from me. I had looked down and seen my arm was still there, all bandaged up. I was filled with happiness knowing I was whole and reassured knowing Gary would only have left the arm if things weren't too bad inside. That made me extra happy.

Once I got back to my room, Mum was waiting for me. She was ecstatic and could not stop talking and telling me I must call people. The only sad thing was that my brother, Allan, wasn't still there. My operation ran longer than expected and he had to leave and get back to the farm. I rang Steve, my boss at Fonterra.

"Steve! I made it! I have an arm! It is just so cool! I have a bandaged up arm and leg with drains and lines everywhere, including my jugular!"

"That's really good news, Barbs! You get well soon and take care."

"Tell all the guys at work it went well and that I miss them and will pop in and see all of you as soon as I can."

"You just look after yourself and we will see you when you're up and about."

"Okay, I sure will. See ya soon."

"Sure thing, Barbs. I will ring you tomorrow to see how you're doing okay?"

"Cool."

Man was it nice to be able to smile knowing I survived and had bragging rights to boot. I was willing to sacrifice my arm, but there it was, plain as day, still attached and free of the tumour that had been tormenting me!

Five days later, I was still in the Manukau Super Clinic. It was late in the day, a long busy day—a good day, with friends Mary and Todd dropping by, as well as Anna who brought me the most beautiful flowers. Mum left after spending four days by my side. Mum helped me through those first few days in a way only a mother can. She stayed just a few miles down the road at a hotel and now felt she could return home to Te Awamutu along with my brother.

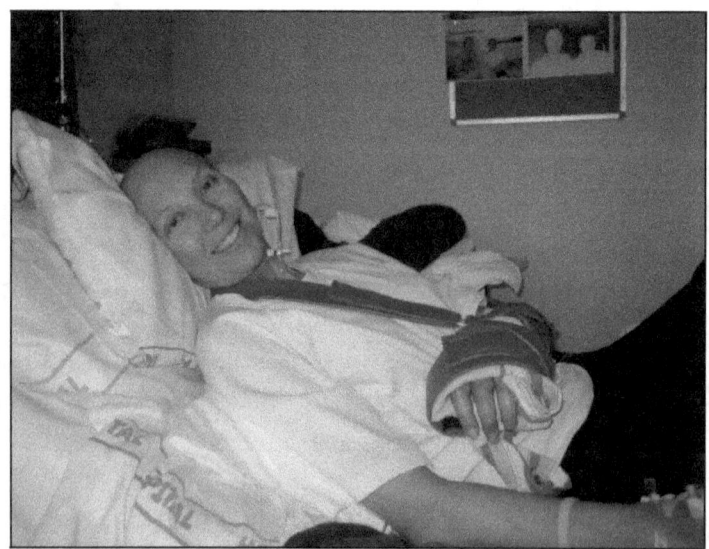

Me at the Super Manukau Hospital, Auckland

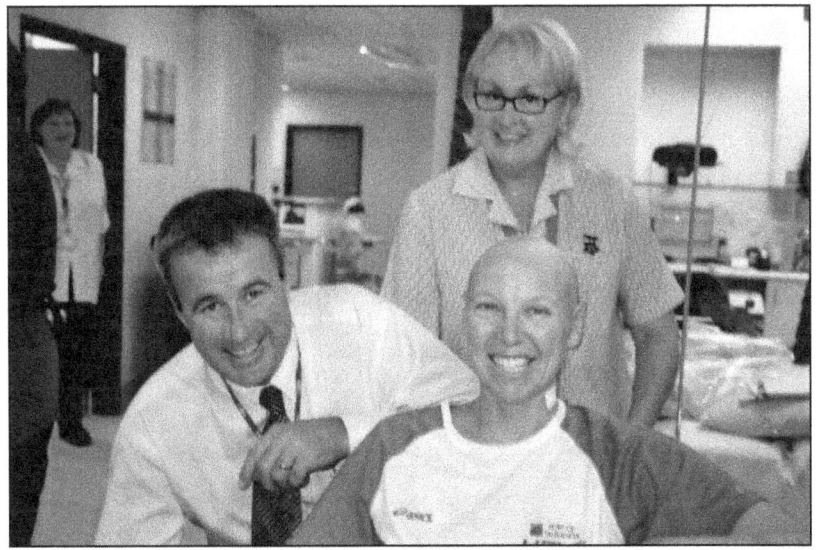

Judith Noonan, Dr Gary French, Karen King and me

I am thinking I have reached a milestone in my journey along the rocky road I am traversing, one wobbly step at a time. I have passed the last buoy in my swim and am turning for home. It was only a few days ago I had every tube imaginable coming out of my body; one tube draining a twenty-five centimetre cut down my leg where Gary removed my fibula—it looked amazing. Ninety percent of the diseased radius and the carpal bones surrounding the cancerous bone had been removed. Now fifteen centimetres of fibula nestled where the radius once was. Some of my fibula remains in my leg to act as donor tissue should I need it in the future—my biological spare part. Along with the drainage tubes were IVs. One was lodged in my right wrist with another in the external jugular vein on the left side of my neck. Once again, my veins were difficult and the anaesthetist was not successful on his first insertion. This is almost unheard of. I wish my oncologist had been there to witness this, as she says my veins are okay. My difficult veins required my jugular to be cannulated. My jugular was a guaranteed hit. Just as well that line had been inserted when I was unconscious! There was also a line with local anaesthetic dripping 24/7 onto the nerves that reached

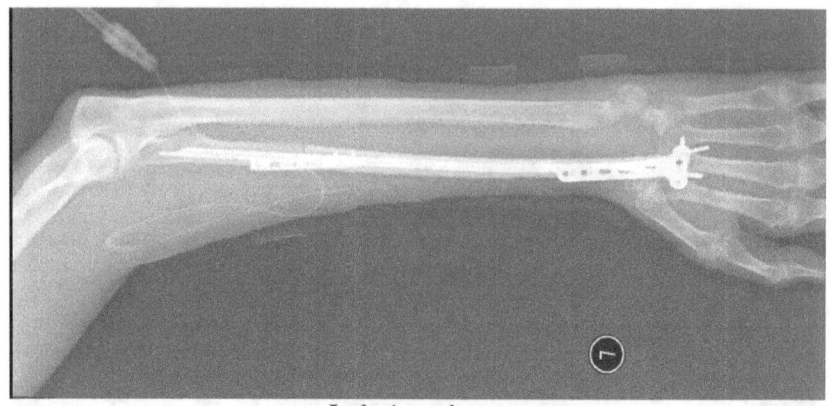

Left Arm after surgery

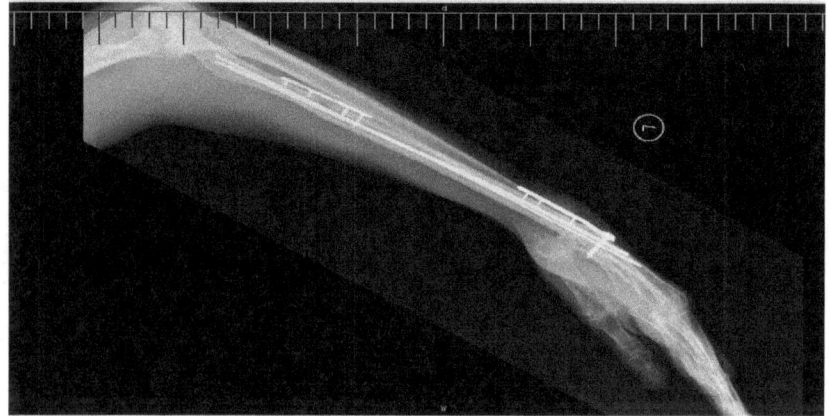

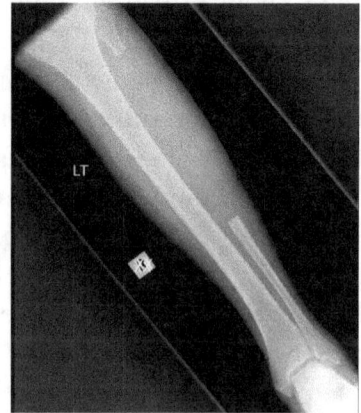

Left leg below after surgery

right down to my fingertips, so I had absolute numbness in the left arm. This line was inserted under my left armpit. Two days later these tubes were detached, freeing me to hobble around the wards.

During my second week in the hospital, my friends Dave & Joy (also Barbara, but known as Joy which is her middle name. We both have the same first and middle names, so to reduce confusion when we are together) came up to visit and to see if it was possible for me to leave the hospital for a day visit to Sylvia Park—a huge shopping mall in South Auckland with more than two hundred shops and four thousand car parks. Thankfully the nurses gave me the green light and we left the hospital.

Half an hour later we arrived at Sylvia Park. It seemed crazy to be so excited about getting into a car again, but I was. It meant so much to me that Joy and Dave took time from their busy lives and drove two hours from Te Awamutu to see me. We had a great day looking at all the shops and lunching at a pub in the mall. Dave pushed me around the shops in a wheelchair on loan from the shopping centre. To borrow the wheelchair, Joy had to hand over her driver's license for security. When we left, Joy retrieved her license and took me back to the hospital. A day later, she realized she had been given someone else's license by mistake. It was so funny. A couple of days later Joy had her own license back.

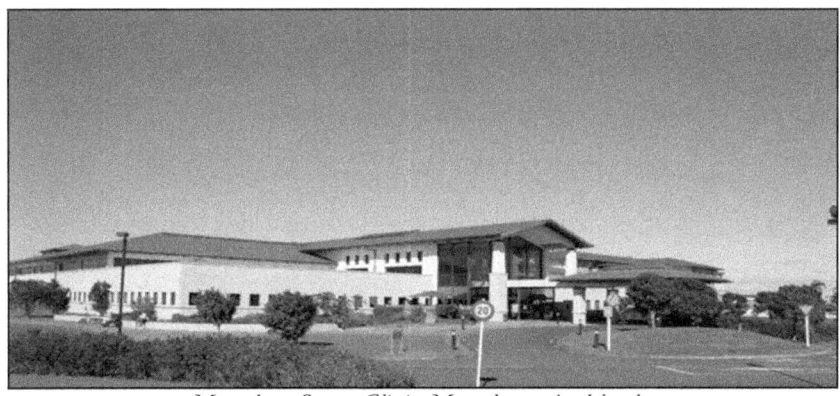

Manukau Super Clinic, Manukau, Auckland

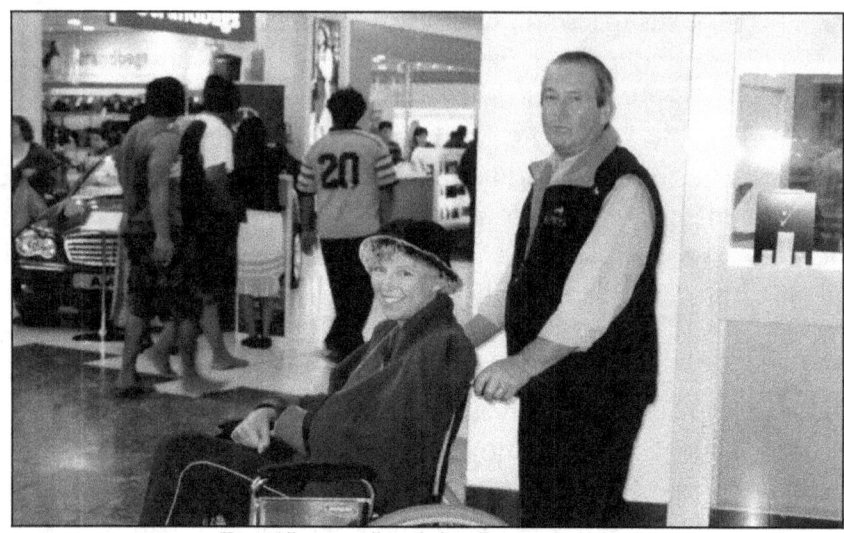

David Lee and I at Sylvia Park, Auckland

More Chemo And Bruce

Cycle Four, June 6-9, 2007. Just shy of four weeks from my surgery, I am on my way back to the hospital for additional chemo and a hot date! In preparation for my weekend, I pack a short skirt, matching waistcoat, white shirt, and black jacket. After closing my bag, I go through the usual ritual of coating my hands with Emla gel and taking my sedative. This time I drive myself to the hospital for the dreaded chemo.

As I unpacked my bag, put my photos on the wall and laid my red blanket on the hospital bed, I told the nurses about the blind date I had arranged. They were excited for me and wanted details. Eager to help, the nurses organized the doctor on duty to have all my discharge papers typed up and ready so I could get away by lunchtime. The nurses are just so cool.

Looking back, I imagined Renée Zellweger or Julia Roberts starring in my role. Okay, I know I took some liberties, but I felt entitled to act as casting director in my own movie, *Chemo Diaries*.

The setting is Ward 25 of the chemo ward where I sit on my bed worrying myself sick, wondering whether my doctors will authorize my discharge. Tonight is my big weekend date with Bruce from Australia. I met Bruce on an on-line internet dating site and after weeks of phone calls and chats, he offered to meet me on his next business trip to New Zealand. As luck would have it, his trip coincided with the scheduled end of my fourth chemo treatment. He purchased his ticket and was on his way. Getting a pass from the hospital depends on my blood test results and more often than not, they have been shockers and I have had to stay in an extra day. Even if my blood tests were acceptable, I often felt so God-awful, there was no way I could leave. The deck was stacked against me, but I was determined to meet Bruce and feel normal again, if only for a few hours.

Looking in the hospital mirror on this, my special date night, I see a swollen face and swollen, bloodshot eyes with dark rings under them. I look like I have gone two rounds with Mike Tyson. I am thinking, "Poor Bruce. He is just not gonna think much of me with this face." I didn't even want to contemplate what he would think of me not looking like my picture. I felt like a fraud, even though I have chatted with him heaps on the phone, mentioning chemo and its ravaging effects, I still felt horrible. Anyway, I made sure the doc gave me some pills to take this fluid off my face by evening—thank goodness they work really fast.

I had prepared for my date by visiting a sexy lingerie shop, buying a sexy bra, knickers and pair of thigh-high stockings. Saturdays in a hospital are on "go slows." There are only one or two doctors making rounds and their day is crammed with visits, consultations and writing all the patient notes. Knowing this, the nurses arranged the House Surgeon to have all my notes typed up the day before so the receptionist just needed to punch a button and they would all be printed. Of course, he was told why and decided this was a great idea and made sure it was all done.

I finally got my good news from the docs. (Told them I was feeling fantastic! Bit of a white lie there, I actually felt awful!) I picked up my discharge notes and flew out the door to my car. It was now approximately 1:00 p.m. My big weekend in Auckland was underway. Bruce was landing in Auckland at 6:30 and told me he had booked the Mecure Hotel with waterfront views in an upgraded suite and had arranged dinner in their restaurant on the top floor. I figured I would have plenty of time to get ready.

I had planned what to wear weeks ago and when I put this outfit on, I struck a major problem. Yes, the "mushy chemo-brain syndrome" had struck again! (I have to point out that this dilemma is worse than a "dumb blond" syndrome. You really do some dumb things! You forget things, leave the stove elements turned on after cooking, and generally stuff up with monotonous regularity!) The outfit I had chosen was a medium short skirt that fit me well ordinarily, but was now uncomfortably tight! I had forgotten about the ghastly eight kilograms I gained from the fluids and chemo pumped into me over the past three days. I was so gutted. I went from 67 kilograms to 75 kilograms in a few days. All of this weight gain without the divine pleasure of naughty sweets or heaps of all those fattening things I would normally have to forgo when trying to stay fit. Lying on the bed, I managed to pull the zip up and that was that, I was wearing my outfit. By now, it was approaching 4:00 p.m. and I figured I would have a relaxed drive to Auckland and wait for Bruce in the hotel reception lounge. At 4:30, I was carefully pulling up my stockings, wearing a fiberglass cast on my left arm, when my mobile phone rang. I forgot all about my cast, reached across my bed for my mobile, and tore a huge, big ladder in my brand new, sexy, thigh-high stockings. Bruce has sent a text letting me know his flight was ahead of schedule and asking me to pick him up earlier than planned. Shit! It's only 4:30 and I am going to have to break the speed limit, as well as buy a new set of stockings!

I decide to stop in Ngaruawahia, buy a cheap pair of "one size fits all" stockings at the service station, and race into their bathroom to change. Being tall, I don't expect these stockings to fit right and of course they don't, but are adequate. Tires screech as I leave the service station and proceed to search the road for someone to follow at breakneck speed, hoping he has a radar detector for cops. Sure enough, just out of Huntly, I find a car driving too fast and tail him all the way to Manukau, saying a silent thanks to him as I take the airport exit lane.

I make it to the airport on time, and present myself to Bruce for the first time ever with no ladders in my one size fits all stockings. I honestly felt like Bridget Jones in all sorts of calamity, but, amazingly, arrived on the scene looking perfect without anyone realizing all the laws I had broken, stockings laddered, and motorists terrorized! I recognized him straight away. He looked as good as he did on the dating website. You don't always recognize blind dates from their photographs—I had learned this the hard way! To top it off, I always made the effort to look sexy as hell, even after three days chemo when I was feeling so nauseated and sick. That really deserved an Academy Award in my book. When I told Bruce all this he laughed, but was in total admiration for my spunk and energy (only God knows where I got it from).

Bruce and I had the most glorious dinner, accompanied by great conversation and laughs. Later, he spent quite a lot of time on his laptop as he had a huge business presentation the next day and I amused myself watching movies.

As the evening came to an end, I was getting quite nervous and still had my wig on. The movie had finished and I figured I'd take my clothes off and get into bed. As I was disrobing, Bruce lifted his head up from his laptop with a smile on his face and gently closed it while still staring at me.

Looking at him I said, "Coming to bed? I am tired, it's been a long day with one thing and another..."

As he placed the laptop on the side table, he walked up to me, put his arms round me and murmured, "You're a brave little thing, aren't you, finishing your chemo this morning, driving up to Auckland, picking me up at the airport, and still looking beautiful." I then thought, gosh, he hasn't seen me with my wig off yet, I am sure I will scare him. If I take it off surely he will walk out and grab the first taxi back to the airport.

"I do like an adventure you know and this sure beats being at home feeling awful on my own. With you, I can forget all that business and enjoy myself."

As Bruce bent down to pull back the sheet for me, he agreed, "That you can, Barbs."

While Bruce was undressing, my wig was driving me crazy. I couldn't stand it any longer and thought it was just too bad if he thought I looked like a freak show, there was no way I could sleep with it on. The look of disbelief on his face only lasted a second, but I could see what he thought. I don't think he will recover from that for quite a while. I really wasn't worried, it felt so nice with the wig off and I just smiled at him. We had sex. Despite my interest in Bruce and great foreplay, it was uncomfortable and unsuccessful. The chemo seemed to have interfered with the way my body worked and I didn't respond at all. I was disappointed and decided to buy some lube tomorrow to make the experience better.

During the night, I had the most outrageous dream that seemed to laugh at my dryness problem. There were flowers everywhere, exotic women in our hotel room and water coming out of the ceiling. It seemed like I was drowning, but everyone else was having a party. I woke up gasping for air. I am getting so tired from the side effects of the chemo. It makes you have ghastly, drugged dreams and you wake up twice as tired and still feeling lousy. Bruce woke up concerned and asked, "You okay?"

"Yeah, just had this awful dream. It was crazy." I sat holding my head in my hands, feeling quite lost. My wig sat forlorn by the bedside.

"Would you like a cup of tea?"

"That would be great." Lying back down on the bed, I watched Bruce go about boiling the jug of water and getting cups out of the cupboard.

"Would you like a lemon tea?"

"Sounds great."

Watching Bruce making tea seemed to relax me and before very long, he put a cup of tea in my hands. The drink settled me down and we soon drifted back to sleep again.

The next morning, Bruce was off to his business meeting and said he would catch up later on in the day. I went downstairs to have breakfast, but I was feeling ill and lost my appetite. I was wearing my wig and all I wanted to do was take it off because I was so hot. Coffee was the only thing I could stomach for breakfast. I needed to get outside in some cool fresh air, but realized, in my hurry to leave Hamilton, I had forgotten my cap and trainers and only had my high heel shoes. This meant shopping. With a new cap I was able to put aside my wig. I splurged a bit and bought a new shirt and jeans. My retail therapy worked wonders and with renewed energy, I set off investigating Queen Street. I bought some lube at a pharmacy and hoped I would get to use it. Sadly, it was not to be. Bruce was busy doing his presentation and arrived back at the hotel for dinner stressed and tired. Perhaps last night had felt as bad for him as it had for me.

I had a glorious weekend in Auckland with Bruce and with great sadness I dropped him off at the airport. You're thinking surely nothing could go wrong now. It is all pretty ho-hum now. Drive home, get over the chemo and carry on. But sorry to say, this story does not end here.

I got lost.

I did read the signs to get back home, honestly. I somehow ended up in East Tamaki or Otara. Chemo and fatigue left me disoriented and my sense of direction just was not working. It took me forty minutes to find State Highway 1 after leaving the airport—unbelievable. All in all, I had a great weekend. I needed to take the risk and it was worth it. Throughout my struggles with cancer, I believe my willingness to sometimes ignore the sensible and reach for a few moments of normality helped me far more than "playing it safe."

Just after my weekend date, the owners of the dating website ran a competition for the best short story about "meeting your website date." I entered and won! Not only did I win, but my friends had a good laugh when I told them. The North Island prize was a white water rafting trip and the South Island prize was a weekend at a lovely hotel resort near Queenstown. I would have liked the weekend at the hotel, however the cost of flying down there, food, and taxis would be huge. In my current state, feeling sick every morning and possessing less energy than a new-born kitten, there was no possible way I could go white water rafting. I sent an email to the website and requested that they give the prize to someone who could enjoy it. They posted me a gift thanking me for my good sportsmanship. The gift arrived a few days later—a beautiful yellow and white striped beach towel.

My "date" gave me occasion to enjoy a moment of being normal again. It is important to take time to "escape" the role of patient. Bruce offered an opportunity to make that escape when I needed it and I am grateful. That was my only date with Bruce. After meeting, we exchanged emails, but they gradually became less frequent and we no longer communicate.

On my next trip to the hospital, I got another plaster cast. Gary took a new set of X-rays that showed my bones were starting to knit. He was extremely happy with my progress. After a series of bright, cheerful casts, I chose black for my new cast to honour the All Blacks & Team NZ. Gary told me the last test result from my tumour and bones had come through. The bones were healing and there was no evidence of cancer outside the margins of the bone that had been cut away. It was the best news ever! I had the best results someone in my predicament could wish for!

If this were television I would wiggle my nose and be cured, but it's not TV and tomorrow I have to return to the hospital for another round of chemo—you know how much I hate this.

Then there will be only one round left to go.

I remembered Bruce's look of horror on seeing me with no hair— well, it was spiky with a quarter inch of hair in patches over my scalp. I decided to get it all shaved off so my head was nice and smooth, just like some guys wear. I chose not to go to a salon and scare the girls, but drove to the end of town where there was a men's barbershop. This was going to be heaps of fun. The part I was looking forward to most was sitting in the barber's chair, leaned right back. As I walked in, I was surprised to find only one guy getting his hair cut. The barber and the client looked round with obvious surprise. "Would it be okay for me to have you shave my hair off?" I asked with a nervous smile.

"Sure. No problem, just take a seat and I won't be long." The barber turned back to his client to finish his cut.

As I was waiting, it felt good to be in a male environment. I did not feel very feminine at all. Before I knew it, I was taking a seat in a wickedly cool barber's chair. It was so comfortable! "Can you shave it like right down to the skin so it is all shiny?"

"Yeah, sure, no problem."

"Cool." That was so much tidier than looking like a ringwormed hedgehog.

"That will be $5.00. Thanks, Ma'am."

Wow, that was almost the cheapest haircut in all my life. How groovy was that?

Walking out the door I felt great; running my hands over my smooth scalp felt nice and relaxing.

Having always enjoyed long hair, I'd never imagined I could feel this way. It was so funny I couldn't stop smiling as I drove home.

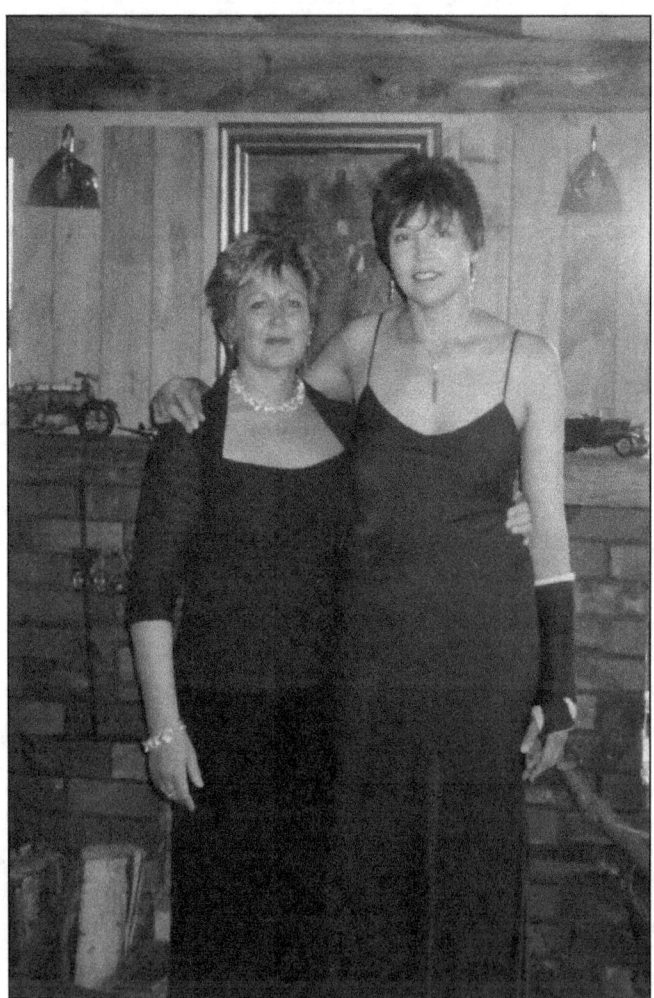

Barbara Lee (Joy) with me and my wig. Going to a Beach wedding party during July at Rings Beach, Coromandel Peninsula

Cycle Five And Mum

Preparing for chemo had become routine. Pack my bag, Emla gel my hands, take sedative, drive to hospital, walk to Ward 25, stow food from home in the patient kitchen, put my photos up, spread my red fur blanket on the bed, set the laptop up, go to the bathroom and run my hands under the hottest water possible. Chris, the Clinical Nurse Manager, would try to put IVs in my poor scarred wrists and we both would hope for the best. Then the horrible sub-cut pump needle would be put into my chest for the antiemetics used to treat the inevitable nausea and vomiting.

On day two of cycle five, I was sick at 6 a.m., but settled by lunchtime.

After the three days of chemo, I drove myself home. Then I did another seven days of GCSF injections into the stomach wall. GCSF stimulates the body's own production of neutrophils by the bone marrow, reducing the likelihood of lethal infections.

During the days that followed chemo, I hoped that I didn't get a cold or become neutropenic and end up back in the hospital again. I became weary of people if they so much as sniffed or sneezed. When meeting people who showed the slightest sign of illness, I took a giant leap back. I was never reluctant to ask those around me if they had a cold.

After chemo, I lose my sense of taste. On day ten, the mouth ulcers start and then I am off my food. Food tastes God-awful and I get no satisfaction from eating anything. Nothing tastes the way it should—tasting worse, much worse, than ashes in my mouth. I want to go to my beach to help me feel better—anything would be nicer than how I felt right after chemo.

During cycle five, I experienced the most difficult two weeks of my life and this time my health was not the culprit. Mum was admitted to the hospital suffering from septicaemia (a potentially lethal blood infection). We all thought she had pneumonia. I raced up to the hospital after the ambulance dropped her off and stayed with her in the emergency department until she was taken to a ward. She answered all the questions the doctor asked her appropriately and I believed she would be released in a couple of days. The septicaemia may have been the result of poor healing from surgery to fuse her ankle twelve months earlier. As with many arthritis sufferers, circulation in the feet is poor and healing after any surgery can be slow. Mum's foot took ages to heal.

The next day, her condition drastically changed and scared the hell out of me. Thank goodness Gael was there helping the doctors make decisions. While Gael was talking to one doctor, another asked us if we wanted to sign a "Do Not Resuscitate" order for Mum. I looked at him strangely and thought, what are you thinking of? How can you ask me that question? I gave him an emphatic "no" and quickly grabbed Gael to reiterate this instruction. I struggled to believe Mum was this ill. It just didn't make sense to me.

Gael was unreal, a tower of strength. I kept thinking, over and over, thank goodness Gael is here, in control, advising doctors and nurses, reassuring Mum, reassuring me. Gael was truly what our family needed in this awful situation. When things really hit rock bottom Gael got us all through, supporting Dad, Allan, his wife, Jan, and me.

Our family camped out in the I.C.U. waiting room that night; every chance we got to see Mum we did. We had to go in one at a time. Mum had tubes and wires stuck to her or coming out of her, as well as a breathing machine, a dialysis machine, and then all of the computers charting her heart rate, blood pressure, temperature and food intake. I just sat there and held Mum's hand telling her, "It will be okay," and any other story I could think of.

Mum went into theatre twice in 24 hours to remove the sepsis from her joints—shoulder, elbow, knees and ankles. She was in the I.C.U. for three days.

July 2007 Last Chemo

Mum had improved and now was in the High Dependency Unit (a step down from the ICU). Our family was having a rough time with both Mum and I in the hospital. When a family feels sure that they cannot cope with another bad thing, something else comes along and they have to find the strength to somehow fight their battles on yet another front. I was so worried about Mum, I was no longer concerned with myself. I still rang the hospital late each night before I went to sleep, so I could settle knowing that she was stable and all the computers connected to her were punching out perfect numbers. Life support was the most frightening thing I have ever witnessed.

As usual, I felt dreadful. My last round of chemo began and I was in the hospital at the same time as Mum, who was fighting for her life in the H.D.U. (High Dependency Unit). My situation was normal, really, as in feeling bloody awful. However, this was the last day I would feel this bad, it could only get better and better! This was my last cycle of chemo!

On day two of chemo I felt so awful, I needed to ask my nurse if I should risk going down to see Mum. It made things a bit easier having Mum only three floors below me. One of the H.D.U. nurses was the daughter of a beach house neighbour. A friendly, known face in a really scary part of the hospital was definitely reassuring. Comfort was taken in knowing there was someone familiar keeping an eye on Mum for us. Pushing my Ivac trolley loaded with fluid, I walked into H.D.U. to see Mum.

I sat in the chair by her bed and just lay my head on her mattress while she was snoozing. A moment later she woke up and said, "Oh, hello." As I lifted my head, Mum gave me her beautiful smile that always made me feel so good and asked, "Hi, how are you doing?"

"Better than yesterday, how are you?"

"Oh you know, I feel like crap, but it is nice being able to pop down and see you. Mum, this is my last cycle of chemo and it's Gael's birthday tomorrow. Do you realize when this all started I came in on Allan's birthday? Talk about coincidental, two dates I won't forget for more than one reason."

"Well, I suppose you'd better head back to your ward so you don't have the nurses growling at you."

"Okay Mum. I am so glad our neighbours' daughter from the beach is in H.D.U. with you to keep you company. It makes me feel better."

"Yeah, it is nice."

"Okay. Mum, I'll drop down tomorrow after I have been discharged and stay longer with you."

"That would be nice, you look after yourself."

"Yip, see ya."

Mum was feeling better today and almost back to her normal self. She was "Mum" again. Last week it was scary, as that sick person connected to the machines wasn't really "Mum."

When I first visited her in H.D.U. she said to me, "Gael will look out for you. You'll be okay." I knew she was saying goodbye, but didn't want to believe she was so ill.

"Mum, you're not going anywhere!"

"Just so you know."

"Mum, you'll be feeding calves before you know it."

"I'm not feeding any bloody calves."

"Good, because you're not going anywhere either. You're gonna be okay."

"I'm not closing my eyes either, so I know I will be still here."

"Oh, Mum," I said, with tears streaming down my cheeks. "You will get better. You have to be around to see me married—God knows when that will be!" We both giggled. Happy that I'd cheered her up, I said good night and told her I would be ringing the hospital every few hours to make sure she was okay.

Being with Mum made it a bit easier to cope with this last cycle of chemo.

There was Mum, connected up to all these machines, and me with an IV bottle of saline/magnesium fluid flushing my body from chemo and feeling like shit. The good thing was Mum and I were able to chat about things and she would soon be out of H.D.U. and into a ward. I was due for another bottle of fluid so I trundled back to Ward 25.

It was so good being discharged from the hospital after my last cycle of chemo. The last thing left to do now was finish the seven days of GCSF injections in my abdominal wall, and then I could relax and enjoy the road to recovery.

I was exceptionally tired, suffering through nausea and forcing myself to eat food that didn't taste the way it ought to. I put on four kilograms in one night that week from all the fluid they pumped into me during chemo, gaining around eight extra kilos in total. I felt so fat and worried I wouldn't fit into my jeans. It might sound crazy in the face of a life-and-death treatment, but sometimes the small things play the heaviest on your mind.

My toenails were all falling off. They went black like someone had dropped a brick on them and before I knew it, my feet were one ugly mess. I counted four black nails: two falling off and two long gone. My fingernails had moons down almost to the tips of my fingers. They were starting to look crooked too. What else was going to happen to me?

Feeling constantly sick is one of the worst things about going through chemo, but there are so many other things that no one tells you about, like, for a constant six months, getting up half a dozen times each night to use the toilet and the resulting sleep deprivation. Sleep all the night through? What was that? I could not remember what that felt like. Food wasn't food or for enjoyment any more. Being tired was something you accepted as normal. I stopped complaining about my lack of energy. Feeling vigorous and lively had become a distant memory.

Blood transfusions—I'd lost count of how many I'd had and one day bought $25 worth of kidney and liver to eat so I wouldn't have to have another one. I would do anything to avoid another stabbing from a 16-gauge needle into a vein that is so pathetic and scarred that the thought of a transfusion seemed to make it shrivel and hide even more.

On top of my woes, Mum had to have her left leg amputated. She knew that if she did not have the surgery she would not get better. The sepsis in her leg was not clearing and the infection leached into her body, causing further illness and stress on her system. She recovered amazingly within a week of the amputation, proving that it was the right thing to do.

Getting myself up to visit Mum daily—feeling sick as a dog, dragging myself up the sodding hill to the hospital doors—wore me out. I had to see her every day or I felt so damn guilty, but I was so nauseated and exhausted. Mum would say, "Don't tire yourself out. You should have stayed home," but how could I do that when the alternative was just lying on a sofa feeling terrible, with no energy and worrying about her. So I got in my car and visited her. Afterwards I felt better, everything seemed okay and I could rest easier.

But soon I would have to really rest, perhaps when I could see real progress with Mum and she was not so fragile—perhaps after another week.

While Mum was in the hospital, Dad took over the daily phone call to make sure I was okay. I found it puzzling at first, a phone call from Dad. To get a phone call from Dad was unusual and I asked him on the first few occasions, "Are you okay? Is everything all right? Has something happened?" I was scared something had gone wrong with Mum.

When I mentioned this to Mum one day, she said, "Dad has taken over my phone calls to you, to make sure you're managing."

I was surprised and humbled at the same time. Mum and I always checked on each other and had daily "Mum/daughter" gossips. It was normal for me to get a phone call from her each day. To get these calls from Dad was truly heartwarming, since a phone call was as rare as a hug from Dad, who loved, but not in a demonstrative way. I had never before felt so conspicuously loved by him.

Recovery Mode

I spent the winter months in recovery mode, celebrating the fact that my chemotherapy was finished, knowing every day could only get better and better. Winter was awful. The cold played merry hell with my arthritis. At least I could sleep in so that most of the frost was gone when I rose. The most irritating part of the past few months was the ever-present cast on my left arm. All my warm clothes have narrow sleeves, which was very frustrating, as they wouldn't pull down over my cast. My favourite silk pyjamas pulled and pilled all down the left-hand side from my cast. I wondered if the cast would ever come off, it seemed to be a permanent fixture. I longed to feel the sun and breeze on my skin. I always chose happy colours; my first cast was pink, then yellow, and then black in support of the All Blacks and Team New Zealand during the America's Cup Regatta. I even cut out a silver fern and pasted it in front of my knuckles to keep up the patriotic theme.

My birthday was in August and I celebrated the end of chemotherapy with my friends at the local Domain restaurant. It was great. I organized a few different groups, as I wanted each party to be small enough to enjoy everyone's company.

I was booked for an echocardiogram at the end of August to make sure the chemotherapy drugs had not damaged my heart. During the test, the doctor said everything looked great. It was brilliant that I didn't have to wait days for the results. Life was looking up. I had another good result from an arm X-ray. I arranged a CT scan of my lungs. I had not had one for ages. This was set for the 3rd of September.

September rolled round and it was time to visit my orthopaedic surgeon, Dr Gary French at the Manukau Super Clinic in Manurewa. I enjoyed these visits, as there was always some improvement with my fibula knitting together with my remaining radius and my knuckles. So great to have positive news, to know my body was progressing well!

The union at the knuckle end with the fibula was taking a while; there was still a gap at the union of the fibula and metacarpals, so Gary wanted my arm to remain in plaster, which meant another joyful colour to choose. Orange. Orange is such a happy, positive and spiritual colour. By now, I could almost do the plaster job by myself. Gary came through with me to the plaster room and I asked if he would mind having his photo taken with me. The nurses all joined in. I always enjoyed a visit with Gary and the nurses at Manukau Super Clinic and took the time to bring them up to speed with my love life and latest website romance. We shared lots of laughter. It was comforting to feel normal and light-hearted around them. Their job usually required them to treat you as someone whose illness had completely disrupted the normal existence most of us take for granted.

Next was a night at Grant's place in Auckland. I'd promised to take him out to dinner almost a year earlier. I had the largest steak that was possible to buy—mmm, simply the best! Even better, I could taste it all!

After our fabulous meal, we got back early enough for me to see the last screening of my favourite program at the time, the Australian TV production *McLeod's Daughters*. I would only watch happy programs, which narrowed the field down to a few shows, and was always glad to lose myself in someone else's little world filled with fun and adventure. During the program I heard a noise in the kitchen and thought it was Grant, but as I turned my head around a different man walked into the lounge.

"Hi, I'm John."

"Hey there, I'm Barbs."

"Going through chemo, huh?"

"No, all finished thank God! My hair will probably take a little while to kick in and grow again, I suppose."

"Yeah, it will. I am just getting another bottle of wine, and heading downstairs. You're welcome to join me if you feel like company."

"Cool, I'll be down soon."

As I watched him walk away, I thought, wow, this is cool, a flatmate at Grant's place. Why didn't he tell me about him? Oh well, not to worry, he was probably just too tired to remember and more interested in dinner.

During one of the ad breaks, I thought to myself, "Oh God! I didn't have my wig on! Oh crap!" He would have seen all the scars on my scalp and forehead where the chemo burned my skin from the inside out. It looked so horrible, like I hadn't cleaned my skin for a week in places. No worries, he didn't seem bothered about it. I am just doing the usual female vanity thing. God knows why! I should be way, way over this by now, but each time some interesting/attractive bloke happened to talk to me, all those same thoughts came into my head, "Shit, what does my hair look like?" And then I'd say to myself, "Well, there is no hair to worry about." Next, "God, the clothes I am wearing look terrible." Those thoughts just seemed to happen automatically.

When I got downstairs, it felt like I had walked into a different house. It was an open plan basement. In the right corner there was a bed, surrounded by green, glass threaded beads from ceiling to floor that divided a foot of white silk. To my left was a bar-kitchen leading to a bathroom. Ahead of me was the lounge part of John's room. To the left was the sofa and opposite the sofa was the stereo and Henry, the miniature rocking elephant. John had found it in pieces in a dump in China. John poured me a glass of Wolf Blass Shiraz and I sat on the floor cushions next to him. Amy Winehouse was playing on the stereo and a mellow mood settled over us. While taking a sip of wine, I casually rubbed my head. I had gotten into the habit of rubbing my head. It felt nice, as it was so smooth now—weird as that sounds—and it relaxed me.

"I miss that. I used to like rubbing my head as well."

"What? How come you had a bald head?" John looked in perfect health and had a number one shaved haircut.

"I had cancer a couple of years ago, a tumour the size of a

grapefruit in my stomach. I was told it was one of the worst cases they had ever come across and things did not look great for me, but they got it all. Went through the most God-awful time."

"God, I have gone through absolute hell as well!"

After we swapped notes and commiserated with each other it was time to hit the sack. I said good night and made my way to the sofa in the lounge, with the gas heater going and a nice cosy blanket and pillow. I fell asleep wearing a smile. It was so nice spending time with someone who had also been there and done that, and whose compassion was unquestionably genuine. It was comforting to see another cancer survivor looking so damn healthy and normal!

My September 11

After a brief unsuccessful call to my GP asking about my CT results, I began to think the news would not be good. I went into the hospital the next day and tried to speak to someone about them. Finally, a doctor saw me but was unable to tell me much at all, so I left feeling even worse.

When my September appointment with the oncologist arrived, Gael, her boyfriend, Kelly, and my mate, Joy, came with me for support. My normal optimism had faded and I sensed the news was going to be bad. Sitting in the doctor's small office, the four of us waited to hear the outcome. Our wait ended when the oncologist arrived and announced, "It is not good news, I am afraid. You have nodules throughout your lungs. They are resistant to chemotherapy and inoperable. Radiation therapy is not an option either as the nodules are too widespread throughout your lungs. Do you want to know your odds, percentage of survival or estimated time left?"

"No, no and no!" I bent my head and rested it in the palm of my hands.

What a terrible coincidence to be told something this awful on September 11th. I left the rest of the consultation to my sister. I could not think anymore. With closed eyes I just kept seeing a black concrete wall I could not climb, change or remove. I did not have any control in what I could see no matter how I tried. Gael held it together incredibly well, despite feeling just as devastated and sick in the guts as me.

What can you say when you hear, "There is no cure?" I know adversity is supposed to make the strong stronger, but at a time like this I think most people become overwhelmed and lost in a reality they want no part of.

The oncologist was not able to confirm categorically that the nodules were cancerous, but all of the other oncologists at Waikato Hospital were of the belief that things were not good. She said she would contact palliative care—I struggled to say this word and refused to think about it. Gael asked heaps of direct questions, cutting through all the nonsense. Joy was appalled at the way my oncologist presented this information to me and was totally pissed off at her.

We left her office. Joy went back to work and said to ring her anytime I wanted a chat and that she would ring me later. Gael, Kelly and I went to see Mum on the orthopaedic ward. She was on Ward 6, where by now the nurses are almost like family, as Mum had been a patient there quite a lot in the past three years and I'd had my brief stint in December followed by Mum once again. Despite her fragile condition, Mum was getting over her amputation and infected joints and was healthier than me. I walked to the ward like a zombie, wanting to stick close to Kelly and Gael and not look anyone in the eye.

I said to Gael, "I just can't tell Mum this news, I can't bear to see the tears in her eyes."

Kelly kept me company and we stayed in the foyer by the lifts while Gael went to see Mum—I felt so guilty not going in with her. Sitting in the foyer with Kelly, I said, "This is stupid, I gotta see Mum."

Kelly murmured, "Yeah, you should."

We went through the doors and up the corridor to see Mum. She had a beautiful smile on her face, but I could see her teary eyes.

"Hi, Mum. It's going be okay. I am going to beat this and not believe the nonsense I have been told. I am going to get better."

"That's right!" Through her tears, Mum agreed wholeheartedly.

"Are they giving you plenty of painkillers?"

"Yeah, I am in no pain."

"Brilliant. It is good seeing you looking so much better."

"Well, we better get going and let you rest. We will ring you later. Is there anything you need?" Gael asked.

"Yeah, I need some more Sudoku books if you remember." Mum

leaned over and showed us the kind of books she wanted.

As Gael, Kelly and I walked out of the hospital, I felt a lot better that I had seen Mum and assured her that I would beat the cancer. I knew Mum—I knew she was crying from the news I had just given her. Despite the devastating news from my oncologist, I was more worried about Mum than myself.

On the way home with Gael and Kelly, a zillion things went through my head, like my whole life was being extracted from a zipped file. All the memorable things I would miss, all the places yet to see in the world and the new experiences to be had. Reeling my mind back to the now, all I wanted was to be with Gael and Kelly and not leave their side—to not be on my own, to be always in their company. I wanted to shut myself away from the whole world except for Gael and Kelly and not see anyone or go anywhere, just live in a cocoon under their protective shield. As the day came to an end, Gael and Kelly retired for the night while I stayed on the sofa watching DVDs. As Gael walked to her room she turned and said, "Watch DVDs for as long as you like. It's okay."

I looked at her for what seemed like a long time and smiled and said, "That's cool. I probably will."

"Wake me up any time if you want to chat."

"Sure."

After Gael went to her room, I watched the end of *G.I. Jane*, which always picked me up a bit. I love stories that end well. I climbed into bed with a book I'd been really enjoying. I wasn't looking forward to closing my eyes and turning out the light as I finished my book in bed. I didn't want to see the darkness. Gael lived out in the countryside and there were no streetlights to lighten the darkness of the bedroom; it's pitch black when the lights go out. Lovely if you want to look at the stars—terrible if your mind keeps conjuring up thoughts of eternal darkness. I decided to keep reading till I couldn't keep my eyes open anymore and then just leave the light on, like my seven-year-old nephew, Jack, does. I didn't want to see any monsters either. Jack, like me, takes ages to get to sleep at night. His mum, Jan, has resigned herself to the fact that it is a family trait. My grandmother used to give me dark looks when she babysat Gael, Allan and me as kids. I was always awake and had to pretend to be asleep to placate her.

I tried to read a book by Lee Child, one of my favourite authors, and struggled to keep up with the storyline. The words became random sentences that made nonsensical paragraphs. Word after word the story was just not sinking in. Scanning page after page of my book with unseeing eyes, endless thoughts zipped through my mind: Mum in the hospital, Dad alone at home, Allan and Jan, my nephew and nieces—Jack, Samara and Patyn—and the possible futures they would have, how beautiful Allan and Jan's wedding was, all our family Christmases, all the good times our family has had together and hoped to continue having… God, I have to get my mind back to Jack Reacher land and see what damage he is up to.

One thing I did resolve to myself: I am going get today over and done with and wake up with a strategy for fighting! I am going to call on my friend the Ironman and take some of his legendary strength into this new fight!

Action Plan

I firmly believe that when faced with something as overwhelming as death delivered to you on a platter, focusing on a plan of action gives you personal power, which goes a long way in restoring a positive attitude. The feeling that you are doomed can stop you in your tracks and is made worse by healthcare professionals who put patients in boxes labelled as hopeless, as terminal. I wanted nothing to do with that label and made sure I surrounded myself with people offering hope and encouragement. I knew staying optimistic was necessary if I was to survive.

I was determined to develop a plan of recovery and the next day I rang some old friends, Philip and Marguerette, to see what they thought I should do. They referred me to a woman who sold a nutritional product that might help me beat this new phase in my cancer. I was no longer fighting a rogue lump in a bone—the tumour had gone viral on me and a whole new plan was needed. I rang my friend, Tom, who is a G.P. and was my personal trainer at Les Mills for three years. He was more knowledgeable about sports health and medicine than anyone I knew. Tom would point me in the right direction and advise me on a plan of action. His friend, Lynne, knew more than most people about nutrition and imported a product that might help. Tom then went through a number of other things I could add to my arsenal. The advice made me feel better. I was starting to gain a sense of control and a plan of action was forming in my head.

Ringing Mum in the hospital was the next thing I had to do. I wanted to let her know I was feeling focused and had a plan and see what she thought of my ideas. I always rang Mum about any momentous decision. When buying my house a couple of years ago, I had to get Mum's approval—then no one else in the family could dispute the decision.

My family does not hold back their views or opinions on things, which always leads to excellent "discussions" around the dinner table at birthdays or Christmases. "Discussions" is the word my family uses, but any stranger would think they were walking into a room where an all-out battle is taking place. To win a "discussion" in our family you need to be six moves ahead of your opponent and armed with facts to back yourself up. Mum ends up being the mediator in a lot of our discussions, therefore Mum's approval has always been important to me. Should any dispute take place later on, I could always finish with, "Mum said it was okay," which always shuts the others up nicely.

After talking to Mum, I took into consideration what Philip and Marguerette and Tom and Lynne had told me, then made my decision to follow Tom's plan and take the glyconutrients recommended by Lynne.

With that sorted, I tackled the practical problems facing me, like work: Income Protection Policy versus a Work and Income Sickness Benefit. A plan is always so helpful and empowering. A plan gives steps to follow, boxes to tick, a course to steer by.

I was due to go back to work at the end of September. With this latest news, there was no way I was mentally capable of focusing on work. I needed to see my boss, Steve, tell him my awful news and ask what would happen to my job. I did not feel able to do this by myself, so once more I enlisted Gael's help.

The next day, she and I drove to see Steve to discuss my situation based on the news I received on the 11th of September. I asked Gael to speak on my behalf as I just could not bring myself to discuss what the oncologist told me that horrible day. I honestly don't know how I would have gotten through that meeting with Steve, Ruku and the HR representatives on my own. I think I would have been a mess and nothing constructive would have been achieved. Gael matter-of-factly told them what the oncologist had told us and breezed through the discussions. She told them I was in no shape to continue working and needed time to focus on getting

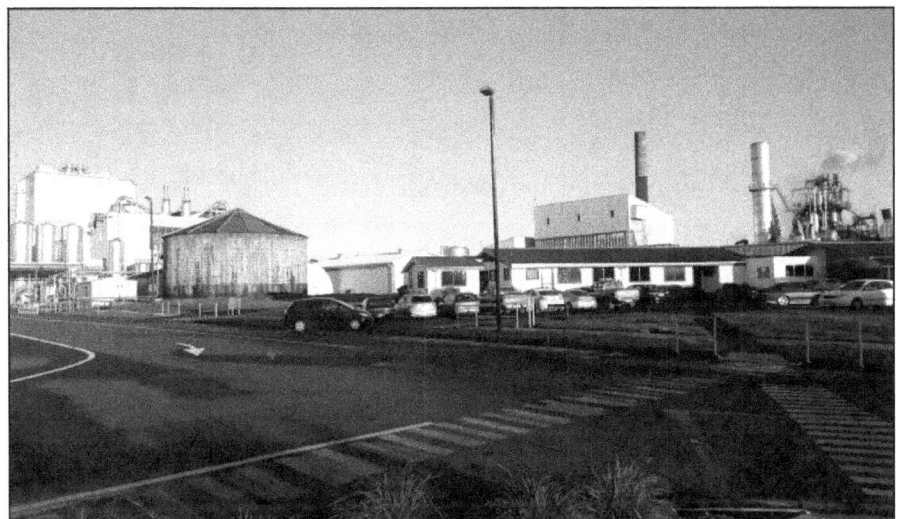

Fonterra - Te Rapa, Hamilton – where I worked   (photo by Jay Baker)

well. At the end of the meeting, Steve walked with Gael and me to our car, just gave me a big hug and said, "You hang in there. You have all of our support. Drop in and have a coffee any time."

The plan that Tom and I put together was simple. Many people would find it unbearable, but I had such enormous faith in the plan because it made sense. I would follow it 100% and would report to my coach, Tom, every step of the way.

I would not get to November 8th—the date of my next scan and the start line for the rest of my life—wishing, "If only I'd done this..." That would be self-defeating and achieve nothing.

I would do everything possible from September the 12th to November the 8th to maximize my chances for wellness. Keeping the plan simple and staying with it was my goal.

My plan included:

1. Organic Vegetables
2. Glyconutrients
3. Reverse Osmosis Water
4. Pure Make-up/Skin Care (or none at all)
5. No Sugar
6. No Meat
7. No Dairy Products
8. Exercise
9. Sunshine
10. Mindfulness
11. Positive Visualization
Friends also suggested:
12. Crystals
13. God

My friend Joy suggested I purchase some crystals at the Pirongia Market, which takes place every year in the last weekend of September. We stopped at a little crystal shop between Te Awamutu and Pirongia on the main road. I loved the colours of the crystals and the jewellery made from them. They were exquisite. That some feel they have healing powers was a bonus for me and I loved the idea. The lady in the shop was fantastic and advised me to get rose quartz for calmness, a bloodstone to help my blood and a few others. Healing powers or not, the crystals were lovely, would not break my bank account and added some sparkle to my plan.

I believed that the bigger the support crew, the better on this journey, and even though I am not a religious person, I asked God along to keep me company as well.

I would carry-out the specifics of my plan in the following manner:

1.   **Organic, alkaline vegetables**. I was determined to get the best quality vegetables with the proper pH level. I went to our local Village Organics shop in Frankton, a suburb of Hamilton. Phil, who

worked there, gave me a food chart that had all the vegetables, fruits, nuts, grains, oils, herbs and spices with their pH listed. I would only eat food from pH 4.0 (neutral) through pH 7.5 (extremely alkaline). The rationale for this was that some research suggested that cancer thrived in an acidic environment. I asked poor Phil so many times to assure me that everything I bought had a neutral or alkaline pH. I only ate broccoli, cauliflower, carrots, onions, kumara, spinach, silver beet, cabbage, lettuce, beetroot, dates, figs, raisins, currants, almonds, avocado and dried coconut, so I could swap from a salad to steamed veggies. These were all organic, as well. I constantly looked at this chart to make sure all of the foods I ate were alkaline.

2.   **Glyconutrients.** Lynne sourced these products from America for me. They were expensive, yet, despite my very bleak financial situation, I had a big enough overdraft to get me started and would worry about balancing the books later. Lynne gave me instructions on how many tablets to take how often throughout the day. I started off at a low level and then increased it in increments to the maximum level Lynne advised. I took tablets four times a day combined with a shake. I invested thousands of dollars in this product. I know the use of glyconutrients to treat cancer is controversial and not without detractors and critics. I am not endorsing the use of glyconutrients in treating disease nor recommending them for others, but I chose to use them and fully committed myself to making these supplements a part of my recovery plan.

It just makes sense to have healthy cells to fight bad cells and the good cells create armies to attack the bad cells. My logic is that each healthy cell that looks like an oak tree under a microscope, multiplied by 600 trillion, is the ultimate defence. As soon as I started this regime I was able to relax a little bit, as I felt I was doing something very positive and powerful to knock the socks off the parasite in my lungs. If you wish to know what brand I used send me an email from my website www.trisurvivor.nz

3.   **Reverse Osmosis.** I installed a reverse osmosis water purification system under my sink ($1000 odd) so I would only drink the purest, cleanest water. This unit takes out every impurity and chemical in the water and is nice and soft and clean to drink. That sounds weird, but drinking water with chlorine in it tastes harsh and metallic and just tainted in comparison. I reasoned that chemical free water would help my cells grow strong and help cleanse my body of all that ghastly chemo. I drank up to four litres a day to help soothe my kidneys, eradicate the dehydrating effects of chemo from my system, and help my damaged kidneys function better. My next goal was to lower my creatinine levels.

The creatinine blood test is used to evaluate kidney and other major organ functions. Each week I prayed for my creatinine levels to go down to normal—100 or lower. My blood tests were like a yo-yo, one week the creatinine was high and the next week it was low. The levels would go something like 169, 160, 167, which was frustrating, but at least the highest level was almost always a bit lower than the previous highest. Sometimes, out of nowhere, it would spike, and I would start all over again. Cisplatin did the damage to my kidneys and I was made well aware of this before they gave it to me. I felt I had no choice believing that if I had not had the Cisplatin, the tumour would not have been killed. I just took a leap of faith and hoped it did not injure my kidneys too severely. My optimism about my kidneys healing themselves was huge. Even though they aren't known to re-grow or heal like your liver does, I decided they would because I wanted them to.

4.   **Make-up/Skin Care.** This step included eliminating questionable chemicals. I emptied all my make-up, moisturizers, deodorants, shampoo, conditioners, perfume, lipstick and eye shadow; everything I put on my skin that wasn't organic was thrown in a box to worry about later. There were beautiful alternatives, but I did struggle finding make-up and just decided not to worry about it.

5.   **Sugar.** Eliminating sugar had to be one of the hardest things to do, as I have a terribly sweet tooth. I usually had two sugars in a cup of coffee (on bad day I would have three) and absolutely loved chocolate. Striking this from my diet was tough, but to starve the cancer cells of one of their favourite foods made the decision easy. I believe cancer thrives in an acidic environment. There was no way I was going to consume sugar for that simple reason. Eating out or accepting food offered by friends and family required me to ask if it was prepared with sugar.

6.   **Red Meat, Pork and Chicken.** Since I was raised on a farm, meat was one of the other things I found hard to give up. My whole diet was based on meat; roasts and steaks were my favourites. Going to my friends' place for barbeques was particularly enjoyable. My new plan didn't stop me from enjoying a barbeque; I just brought along a salmon steak wrapped in two layers of tinfoil to protect the delicate meat from the carcinogens in the flames. Other guests often envied my meat choice at barbeques.

7.   **Dairy Products.** This was another tough one for a farm girl. I remembered the times we would go to the beach with milk from our cows in a three-litre jar and after three hours travelling it would be 50% cream, which Mum poured over hot apple pie when we got there. I loved milk, and cheese cooked and melted in all imaginable ways. Again, the rationale behind not eating dairy was increased acidity levels in the body when consumed. There was no way I was going to give the cancer in my body any chance to survive. I would starve it to death!

8.   **Exercise.** This was the most enjoyable part of my regime and it kept me focused. My friend, Tom, wrote a program up for me and kept me motivated, along with some personal training at his gym. It took me back to my Ironman training plans. Most of my exercises were based on core muscle strength, as I wanted to keep up my triathlon fitness. One thing about triathlon is that to swim, cycle and run (or walk) comfortably requires a good core muscle base. One day, I will cross a triathlon finish line, be it a beginners' 300 meter swim, 9 kilometre bike, 3 kilometre run or a full Ironman. Exercise was essential.

9.   Sunshine. This was something I looked forward to everyday and by now the weather was improving; spring was being kind to us and nice, sunny days were frequent, which helped this part of my recuperation. Tom said to get as much sun as possible in the late afternoons when it was safe to be outside with no lotion. Since I loved the sunshine, I decided to change this. I sunbathed in the middle of the day when the sun was at its warmest, but only for fifteen minutes each side. As I have olive skin, I was more tolerant and always went brown the next day. Since I hated tan lines, I decided to find a secluded spot of my back garden to sunbathe nude. I found a place in the corner of my garden, which was fenced and surrounded by shrubs and let sunshine in at the corner of my house. I checked that there were no flight paths over me, then put the radio on, set the alarm on my mobile phone for fifteen minutes and snoozed naked on a lounger. The sun warming my bones and body was so nice and I was getting a great suntan. Tom told me there is good scientific evidence that the sun can help fight off cancer—like many things, a little bit is good for you.

10.   Mindfulness. Tom also suggested listening to CDs by Jon Kabat-Zinn first thing in the morning and last thing at night before I slept. I wasn't sure if it would work, but because it made sense to de-stress the mind to facilitate everything else in day-to-day life, I took it on board. This was my meditation. It was all positive stuff; therefore it could only be good for me.

11.   Visualization. Two researchers in Australia made a documentary about the pollen of certain flowers, which, when injected into a cancer cell, exploded it to smithereens. The digital movie of this was fantastic. I cannot remember when this played on

TV, but having previously seen the process, I visualized it myself for each cancerous nodule in my lungs. When I was driving somewhere or sitting at home watching TV (or at any time) I visualized my cancerous nodules being injected with this pollen and annihilated into dust particles, then eaten up by an army of white scavengers and natural killer cells in my body. I visualized the scavenger army and killer cells being made stronger by the glyconutrients I was taking. I also visualized each of my healthy cells as a tyrannosaurus hunting the cancer cells down and devouring them.

12.   Crystals. Joy has a large crystal rock on her table, which is just beautiful, and she explained to me that some crystals have healing powers. I decided why not try them! Mostly, they looked so pretty and the jewellery made from them is gorgeous. It was nice to wear beautiful crystals day and night and let them do their work. Even if this was a bit "out there," it didn't matter, it was just another piece of the healing puzzle that might help.

13.   God. I think I went to Sunday school twice when I was a kid and while under the age of ten, I attended church once or twice when staying with a friend. I decided to invite God on this journey as well. Not that I knew a lot about him. I just figured one could never have too large a support crew in this world. I was in such a vulnerable place and so scared that every time I went to Lynne's place to collect my glyconutrient products, I would ask her to say a prayer for me and ask for God's help.

Just A Bit Busy

My Auckland orthopaedic surgeon, Dr French, encouraged me and helped me stay positive when he told me the lung nodules did not make sense. I agreed. However, a tiny bit of me believed what the X-rays said. My lungs were covered in tiny nodules which were chemo-resistant, inoperable, too widespread for radiation and too small for a fine needle aspirate biopsy.

I am not going to let those little buggers stay long enough to do their worst! I am gonna get rid of them one by one! If I have to visualize each one being bombed with a grenade and exploding into nothing, then I will do it, along with everything else!

The crux of it all was that no one knew for sure. The fact remained that my oncologist had handed me over to palliative care and was not very encouraging. There had been a case-conference held at Waikato Hospital attended by every oncologist on staff—all agreed that there were no further options for me except palliative care.

My follow up CT scan was booked for November the 8th. I scheduled the scan on the luckiest day of the month. In the Chinese world, eight is a very lucky number. Being the positive person I am, I see this as a good omen. I believe I will have the best result, despite what those very qualified doctors thought.

Each weekend I stayed at Joy and Dave's place. Weekends were the hardest to get through, as during the week I kept pretty busy, seeing Mum, doing odd jobs and completing my little exercise regime. There was always something to do during the week.

Joy suffers from Crohn's Disease and has had a rough time of it in the past few years. She came close to dying a few years back. Her incredible fortitude is simply amazing. Joy is honest and always tells it how it is. She has the largest heart and would move heaven and earth for someone in strife. Joy has instant, witty answers for any cheeky comments made, where I always end up thinking of a witty answer the next day. Dave is a typical Kiwi bloke, with his head under the bonnet of a car, fixing up an old motorbike in his shed, or tweaking his distilling unit that makes gin or whiskey. Dave is a salt of the earth kind of guy and has a "spade's a spade" personality. Watching *Top Gear* on TV with him was always a highlight of my weekends.

Every Friday night, Joy invented new meals made from the few vegetables I could eat. She created tasty, gourmet meals, which was a real treat, given I took the easy way out and just steamed them. Joy made lovely stuffed kumara, using all the rest of the vegetables as toppings. Another dish was made of layered vegetables, alternating kumara slices with the others as a kind of baked vegetable pie. She did countless other things with my veggies but these two have stayed in my mind. We sarcastically talked about how "sick" I looked. Quite honestly, I felt I looked healthy. I had a nice suntan from my daily, full-body, thirty minute bake. My physical fitness had improved from weekly training with Tom in his office. Joy and I had a good laugh about me looking "sick" because she certainly didn't believe I looked like I was going to die.

One nice, sunny day I was sitting in Joy's garden on a sun chair reading and heard her say through her kitchen window, "Have you rung your Mum and Dad yet?"

"Mmm? I'm just a bit busy at the moment."

"Like hell you are, you lazy miss," she scolded.

It was so nice, swinging with the sun shining down on me warming me all over. I felt so comfortable I didn't want to move, but I did call Mum and Dad later that day.

Joy's brilliant. She always kept me on my toes and gave no quarter and said what she thought. Most of all, she supported me as much as she could, gave me positive reinforcement and shared her healing surroundings. No negative stuff was allowed. But, in saying that, Joy also encouraged me to get my fears out, as they are better out than in and not half as bad when shared.

Other times, we went to Joy and Dave's good friends' place for a coffee and gossip or went shopping. One weekend we went to the Pirongia Market Fair. Craftspeople from around New Zealand arrive in Pirongia every September on market day to sell their wares—it's brilliant for bargains, there's always something different you won't find in shops.

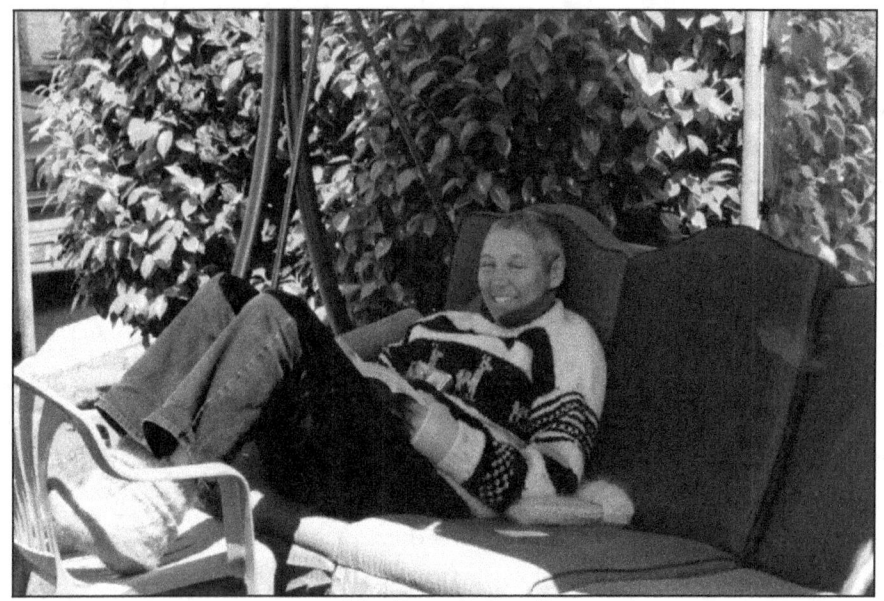

Me, "Just a bit Busy"

It was also a chance to catch up with people we hadn't seen for ages.

Once or twice, we did seriously talk about my cancer, but we both ended up in tears and decided this was not fun and didn't talk about it again. Joy needed to know that I was aware of how serious things were. She didn't want me to be oblivious to the possibility that the cancer could kill me. She didn't want me to cheat myself out of tying up loose ends, saying goodbyes, preparing my mind if the cancer was going to win.

I do know I looked at things differently. Some days as I was driving home or back from the beach or to see my friends in Napier, I'd realize that I live in a very beautiful country. Mostly, sunsets and sunrises started me thinking about this. The beginnings and ends of days are like the beginning and end of our lives.

Being with my nieces and nephew, who are just gorgeous, would make me wonder what they will do for jobs, who they will marry and if I will be around to see them grow into adults.

My family and friends mean the most to me. When I thought of what the oncologist told me, the idea of not being with them hurt so much. Those thoughts went through my mind when I least expected them, invariably when I was having a great time with my family and friends. I would just sit back and look at them for a long time, imagining their futures. On those occasions, I stopped to think and wonder if I would be here in six months time or even the next time my family members laughed, teased each other, or simply shared a barbeque together.

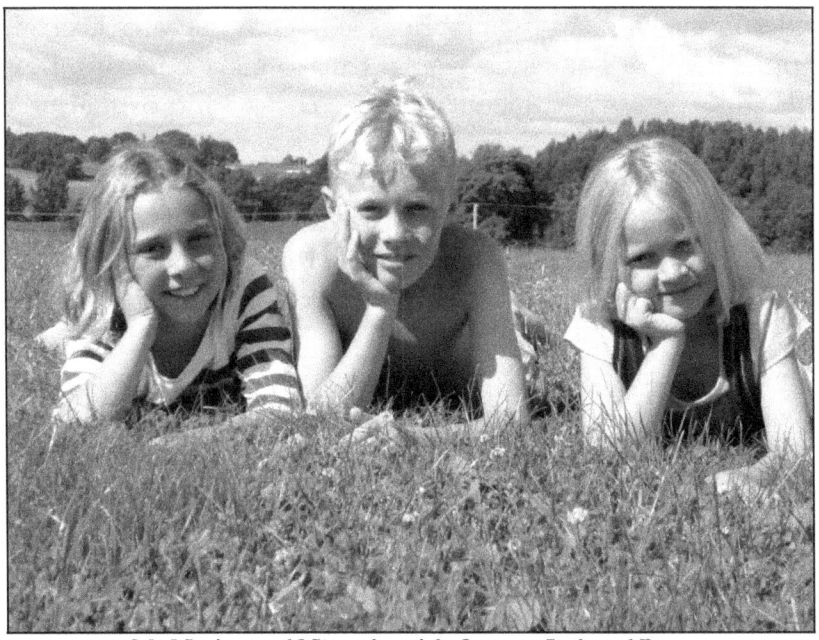

My Nephew and Nieces from left: Samara, Jack and Patyn

Because I refused to be told what my odds were, or the length of time I would have left to live, or the percentages of surviving this cancer, I just enjoyed each moment to its fullest. To me, knowing the odds might mean I would conform to them. I wanted this to be my own race with no outside expectations.

I kept hanging on so I could eventually enjoy the largest steak, rib roast, hot buttered toast with marmalade, and wine! Oh, to be normal! How true vegans have fun is beyond me. After my first month of nothing but vegetables, I felt like I was going crazy. I found the discipline to stay on my diet knowing it would help maintain a neutral pH and a good result. My reward for good behaviour was beetroot, carrot and apple juice. When I felt most deprived of the foods I loved, I would think of the cancer cells slowly starving too—starving, shrinking, being gobbled up by my newly energized immune system.

The most exciting thing I looked forward to was going to the beach near the end of October. The folks on our beach organized a Blender Party where everyone brings along a bottle of vodka, gin or any other spirit or liqueur, as well as fruit to make cocktails. It was a real laugh! There was a blender connected to a motor that used to be a weed-eater.

After the blender was filled up with fruit and alcohol of all descriptions, Steve pulled the cord, started the motor of the blender (like a chainsaw) and let the good times roll. The blender had a rev control to make it blend faster or slower. The noise of a chainsaw making a cocktail was just the funniest thing ever!

While I was at the party I, of course, could not drink any of the cocktails and found that tough, but I knew I would be the only one smiling the next morning. I ended up asking people what their drinks tasted like, requiring them to give me a detailed description. I walked around with a glass of water while they drank their cocktails. I stuck to the plan, and felt like my cancer withered and died inside me.

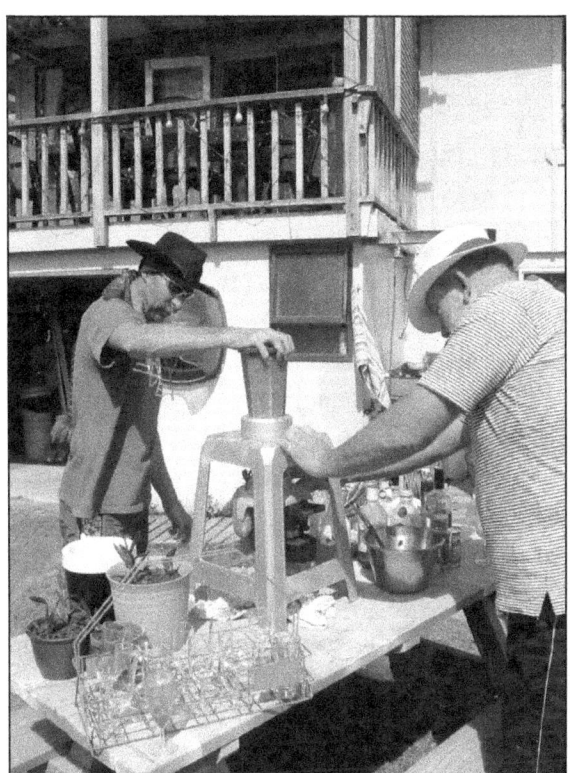

Steve McIntyre and Desmond Tierney
Blending the next cocktail drink

November CT Scan

Feeling a bit nervous with only a few days left until my November 8th CT scan, I increased my glyconutrients to as much as I could afford. One particular product cost $100 per container and I was taking a full container of it each day. It was an integral part of my plan to combat the cancer. This was only possible thanks to Fonterra placing me on special paid leave during my absence from work, then making me medically redundant when I could no longer cope with working.

Lying in the CT scanner, I mentally ticked off all the good things I had done to help my body: eating only the best foods, drinking the cleanest water, moderate sunshine, visualization, no chemicals on my skin, no sugar, no meat, no dairy products, plenty of exercise, meditation, crystals, great friends and family and a positive attitude. During the CT, I offered the longest and most heartfelt prayer to God to please, please give me cancer-free lungs.

The next five days dragged by while I waited for the results. I felt like I was walking around on a tightrope waiting to fall. I want to be around to have great times with my family and friends. I want to see my nephew and nieces grow up.

I rang my coach, Tom, to see if he could be with me when I got the results on the 13th. He said, "Absolutely! I'll be there. I will meet you in the waiting room." Gael and Kelly would drive in from Te Awamutu and Joy would drive me to the appointment. I invited God on the ride. I wonder if God waits for invites or just comes along for every ride regardless.

I needed my support crew with me, as they had all helped so much and each had been an integral part of my recovery plan.

Tom was already in the waiting room when Joy and I arrived. Gael and Kelly arrived next. I was beginning to wonder how we were all going to fit in my oncologist's office as it was so small. I decided it was not my problem. Tom could talk to her in "doctor speak" to clarify what she was saying if I looked glassy-eyed. Gael could rephrase the oncologist's words so I could understand them. I have always struggled with deciphering her. It just might be a personality clash, who knows? Joy could hold my hand and pick out something—anything—positive for me to focus on.

"Barbara?" With a big smile on her face my oncologist motioned me to come in her office. She doesn't usually smile.

"Has everyone got a seat?" my oncologist asked, surprised at the size of my support crew. A chorus of "yes" rang out around her small office.

"Well, Barbara, I can tell you, your news is good. There seem to be no nodules on your lungs anymore. They have gone."

"Wow! Wow, wow, this is so, so cool!" The most amazing, tingly feelings of euphoria, jubilation and happiness shot through me. I smiled so big I thought my face would split. I wanted to shout, "YES!" at the top of my lungs.

While I was revelling in this unbelievable news, the discussion in the room was about my kidneys. Gael asked my oncologist if they would ever get better and if the creatinine levels would go down. My oncologist said, "No, they won't go below 170 or 160. Barb's kidneys have been damaged by the Cisplatin."

I turned round and said with conviction and belief, "Oh yes they will! My creatinine levels are going to get much lower than that!"

If I can cure myself of cancer, I can most definitely get my kidneys to behave themselves. They will get at least 1 litre of water a day to help them recover.

We left my oncologist's office in uncontainable joy at what we had achieved. I can now say to myself what the doctors and nurses could never say to me: I am going to be okay! Make that better than okay! I am going to be well and live!

I immediately rang Mum and told her my awesome news and we shed tears of happiness together. I promised I would drive home to see her and Dad as soon as Joy dropped me off. Next on my call list was my brother, Allan, and Jan, his wife. The joy in their voices was something I won't forget for quite a while. Allan was always there through my most horrible times with chemo. He always made me feel better. He would tell me a fishing story that made me laugh when times were bad. I'll never forget Jan offering to give me blood for my first transfusion.

Next, I called Steve from Fonterra. Steve was in Chicago and he was elated for me. He mentioned to me how cold it was there at the moment and how he was in a bar having a drink and Graeme had just bought him a beer. I so wished I could just wiggle my nose and be in a bar in Chicago with Steve and Graeme to celebrate. But I was in lovely New Zealand and it was lunchtime—time for a cheeky, celebratory glass of wine.

As Joy drove me home, the most appropriate CD was playing: Queen, singing "It's a Beautiful Day." All the way home Joy and I sang along at the top of our lungs. It was so cool. When she turned her car off in my driveway, we just sat there in silence and looked at each other.

A little while into that silence just looking at each other I started to smile, Joy started to smile, and then the widest grinning faces were looking at each other with tears in our eyes followed by a loud, high-pitched, "YAHOO!" from me.

"Joy, I so can't believe it! There just aren't enough words to describe what I am feeling! I want to go crazy with my MasterCard—celebrate and buy whatever I want to!"

"Honey, you have no money left."

"I know. I am gonna have to move out of my house and rent it to cover the mortgage."

"That's a good idea. Will you go and stay at your mum's?"

"Yeah, and save some money and get a new job and get life back to some semblance of normalcy again. But somehow, I am gonna celebrate this news, Joy, and it will be huge and expensive, I know that for sure!"

"Like how?"

"I am going to see my friends overseas to show them that I am still alive and celebrate all around the world. I think I will go to the Farnborough Airshow in England, across to Denmark to Legoland, pop over to France to watch the Tour de France in the French Alps of L'Alpe D'huez, then to Dubai on the way home."

"Sounds great! Pop round for dinner tonight after you have been out to see Mum, Dad, Allan, Jan and the kids. Dave will be glad to hear about your news tonight over a beer."

"Cool. I can't believe it. We've done it!"

"I know!" Joy said with a look of admiration.

"Okay, I'll see ya tonight mate! I really must get home and see Mum and Dad."

"Yip, I'll see ya later."

The rest of the day was a blur of uncontained happiness. Lying in bed that night my face ached from smiling so much. For the first time in months I dared to think of the future, and of all the people who had helped and supported me on my rough, twelve-month journey. How could I ever repay their support?

I will be forever grateful to the sport that brought the tumour to my attention. Triathlon and the daily dedication of training and focus gave me the discipline to follow the new path I was given— the one from cancer to health. Had it not been for the Half Ironman on the 9th of December 2006, I do not believe I would be here to tell you this story.

My inspiration came from watching Ironman in Taupo in 2005. Hearing the "Voice of Ironman," Mike Reilly, saying to every finisher, "You. Are. An. Irrrrroooonnn Man!" will stay with me for a very long, long time.

As sleep slowly claimed me after my most happy day, I drifted off, dreaming that perhaps one day I might hear Mike say to me, "You are an Ironman!" Cos me and Mr. Ironman…. we have unfinished business!

Epilogue

My December 2011 check-up was negative for cancer. I have been given a new beginning and faith that things which may seem unattainable are not out of my reach. This unshakeable belief in my ability to achieve the impossible is a fundamental part of my DNA.

In 2008, I followed through with my extravagant plan to travel around the world. I booked it all on my VISA card with not a cent saved. I am still paying it off—happy I took the leap and splurged!

On my world tour, I visited my friend, Mike, from Dubai, who I originally met at the 2008 Ironman competition. We had stayed in touch through email and on impulse I rearranged my trip to include a stop in Dubai. Being a hot weather gal, I loved the dry heat. He was a gracious host and went out of his way to make sure I enjoyed my stay.

My love of aviation lead me to the Farnborough International Airshow in England, which my Dad went to many years ago before immigrating to New Zealand in 1951. Hearing an F-16 take off was deafening and exhilarating at the same time.

The Tour de France beckoned. There, I made three wonderful new friends: Paul, Carl and Jim. Their delightful sense of humour, love of sport and zest for living made my time with them the highlight of the Tour de France. They encouraged me to write this book and for that I am ever thankful.

My concern for eating right was a constant companion while travelling, but I had no road map to follow, no one to say, "This is what you should eat now." There was no "debriefing," like soldiers have after a nasty mission, to take away all the ghosts and nightmares which follow a harrowing experience. I had to fumble my way through each day saying to myself, "I am okay. Everything will be okay." I was my own coach, continually reminding myself to think twice about everything I ate or put on my skin. Was it in its natural state or processed? Acidic or alkaline? I read every lotion and cosmetic bottle, ensuring no parabens were listed in the ingredients. If the ingredients read like a foreign language, the product was left on the shelf. These habits stayed with me for a long time.

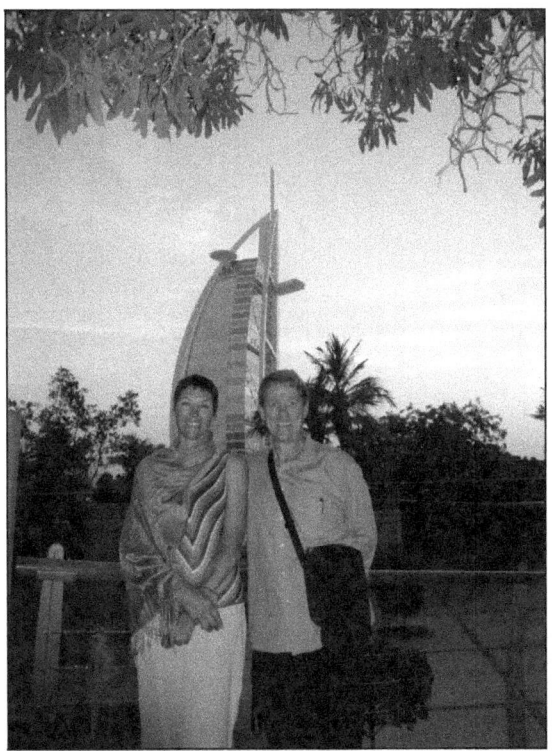

Mike Fooy and I – Dubai 2008

My modified vegetarian diet continued. However, I treated myself to a steak at least once every two months or so. Sugar and milk products were strictly avoided. Glyconutrients were continued, but taken at a maintenance level. These nutrients were my safety net. I decided I had to keep doing what I did during September and October of 2007, keeping my body in an alkaline state. I don't know what worked—what killed the nodules that had metastasized throughout my lungs. It didn't matter. I had achieved the desired result!

After Cisplatin damaged one of my kidneys, I was determined to bring my creatinine level down to normal limits. My oncologist said it was unlikely I would ever get below 167. Normal parameters for a creatinine blood test result are 45–90. Bucking the odds, my kidney function has improved dramatically, with creatinine levels fluctuating between 96 and 125. Now to find a nice, dry, hot place to live and shoo away my arthritis for good!

Fortunately, I have a health insurance policy, because in 2011, joint damage from arthritis required dual knee replacement surgeries. My surgeries were successful and I feel like a baby *Forrest Gump*! In late June of 2011, I could walk without pain in my knees and have been dreaming of doing triathlons again for the first time in four years. Unmet goals are once again within my reach!

In January of 2011, over a coffee with Gael, I learned the doctors had given me 6 months to live when the nodules in my lungs were discovered. I continue to believe that estimates like these can cause unhealthy emotional reactions and I am happy Gael waited until I was healthy before sharing this with me.

During the summer of 2010, I found time to cry. The tears started from embarrassment over something very stupid I did while on holiday at our beach house. The beach beckoned like a friend to heal my wounds and the sea breeze whisked away my troubled, pent-up emotions. The sunset cloaked me in its warmth and gave me the serenity I longed for. Tears of anguish, fear and anger were replaced with tears of joy and gratitude for a life filled with the wonders of my beautiful New Zealand, friends and family.

Today, I am still pinching myself. I am alive and cancer-free! Watching the sunrise each morning is a gift I never take for granted. A few weeks after learning the nodules in my lungs were gone, I had a dream:

I was out fishing with Allan—sitting in his boat thinking what a glorious day we were having in the sunshine—when God rose up over the foredeck. I looked up and said to Him, "Thank you." He gave me the warmest smile and faded into the sunshine.

I know I can always count on my family and friends. Without their support, I would not have gotten through the last few years.

I am now training for triathlons and maybe—just maybe—the ever illusive Mr. Ironman.

Photos

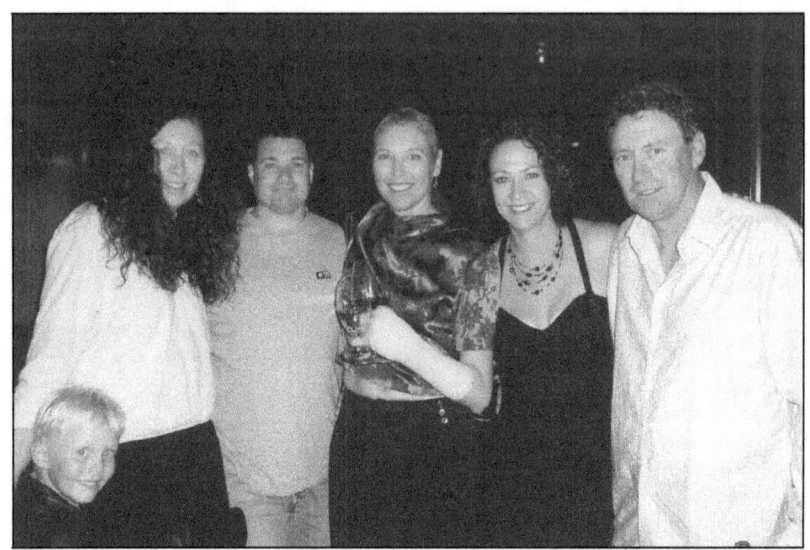

Above: Nephew Jack, Gael, Kelly, me with my lovely yellow cast, Jan and Allan

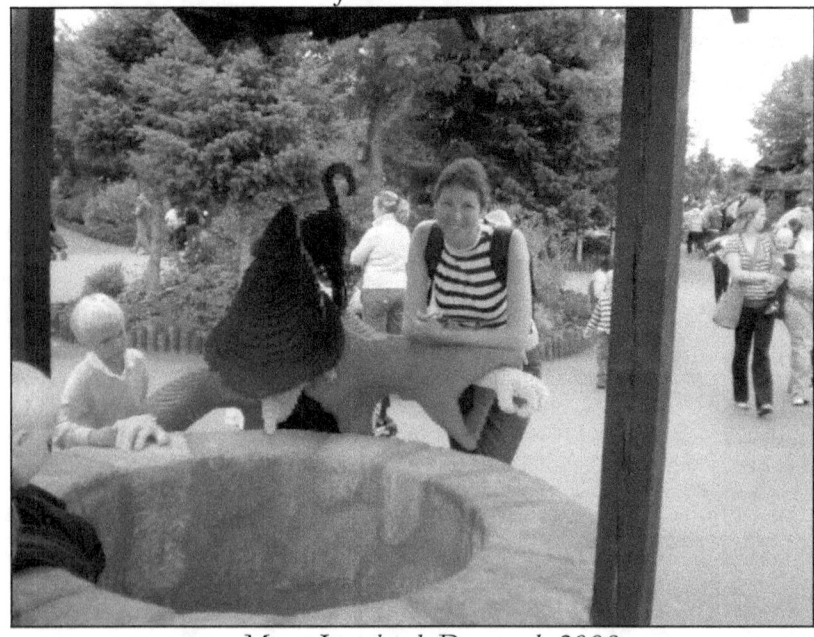

Me at Legoland, Denmark 2008

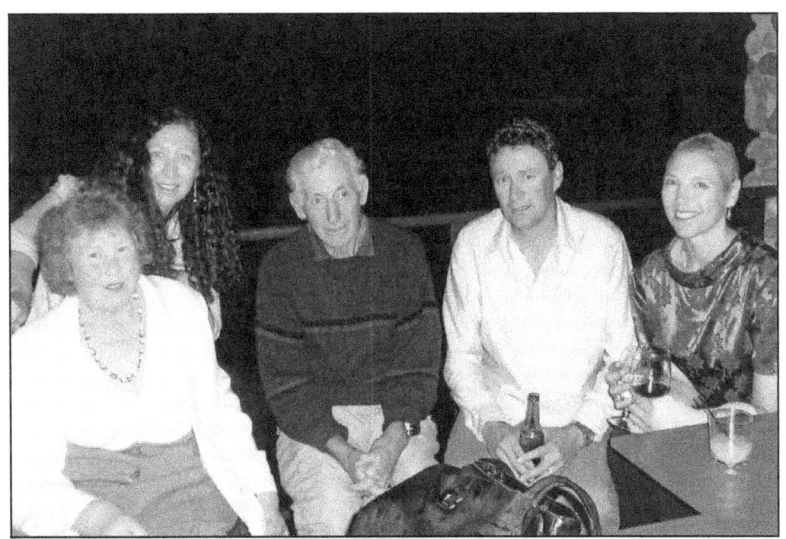

Allan's 40th Birthday: Mum, Gael, Dad, Allan and me

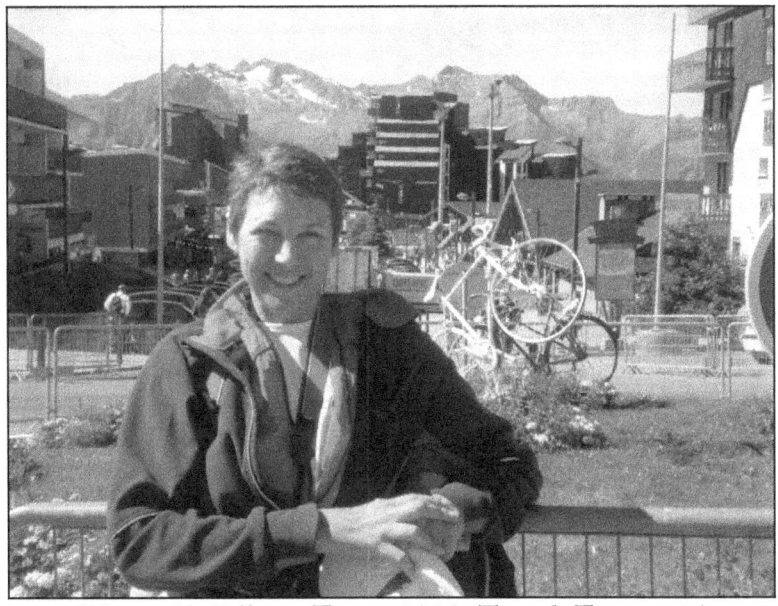

Me at Alp D'huez, France 2008 (Tour de France trip)

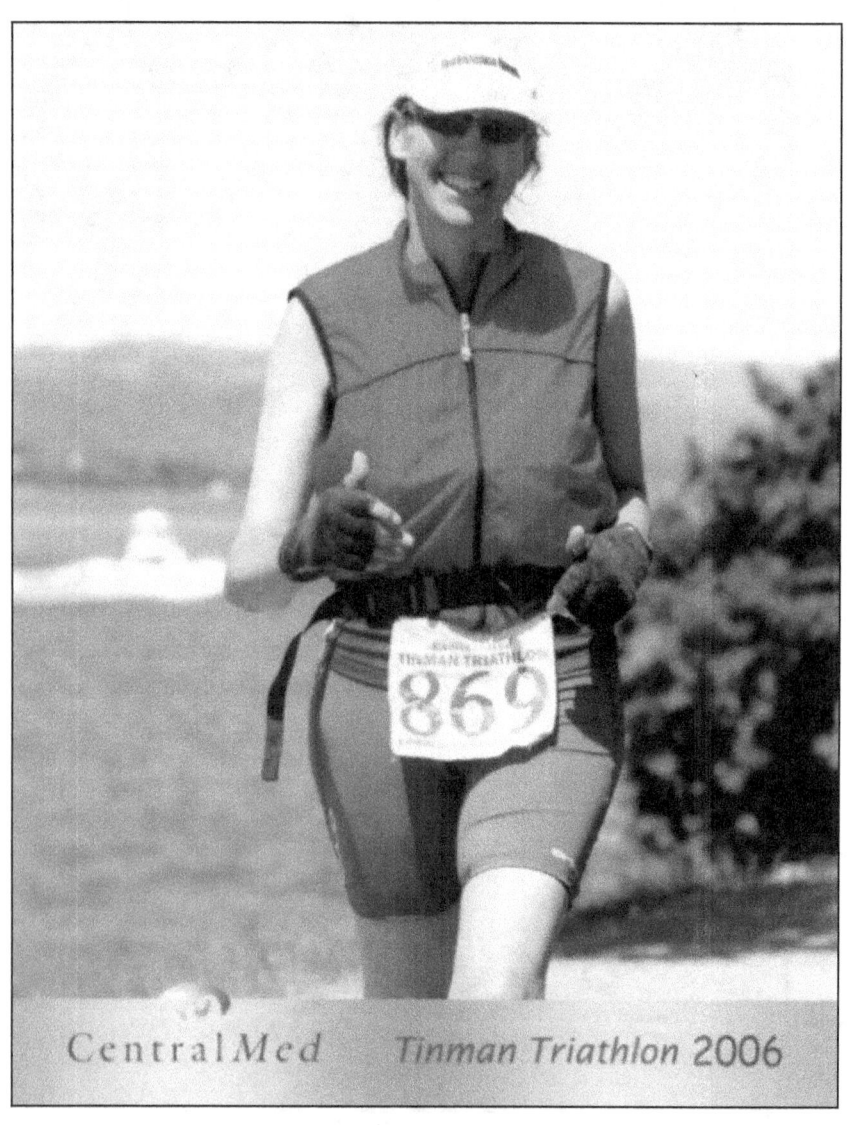

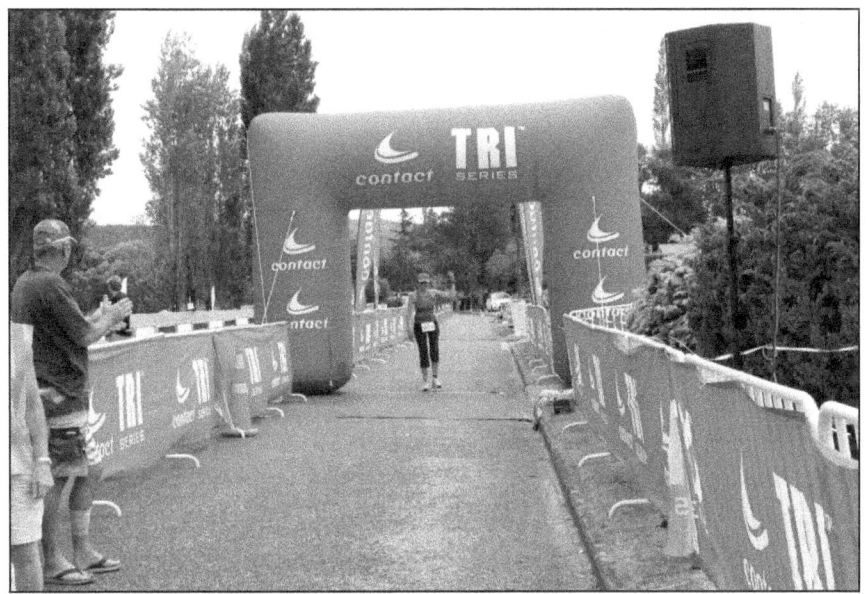

2012 NZ Contact Triathlon, Kinloch – 300m swim : 9km Bike : 3km Run
first and last triathlon since 2006

Have you ever wondered what you would do if an Oncologist told you to get your affairs in order? Would you want to know how long you have left to live? Would you turn to Google for some miracle cure? This story takes you on Barbara's journey facing such questions herself. It is more a personal journal but most importantly how Barbara survived and what she did to overcome secondary cancer against all odds.

———————

Barbara's inspiration is immense. The power of her passion and desire to dispel any fears in her life makes her an Ironman in the truest sense of the word. Through her training and strong mental attitude Barbara has built a road to healing, a road with a finish line just for her!

Mike Reilly
"Voice of Ironman"

———————

Barbara was raised on a farm in Puahue, Waikato, New Zealand. She was diagnosed with rheumatoid arthritis in 1997. In 2005, she discovered Ironman and set a goal to complete Ironman Taupo. In 2007, Barbara was diagnosed with bone cancer. Today, she is cancer-free and sharing her inspirational story.

www.ingramcontent.com/pod-product-compliance
Lightning Source LLC
Chambersburg PA
CBHW072130280526

45788CB00002B/586